HAVING BABIES

From the Wonders of Conception to the Joys of Parenthood

written and edited by
Toula Hatherall
Royal Victoria Hospital, Montreal, Canada

contributing writers:

R. Bresnen • E. Carswell • M. Clement • M. Copp • B. Gillett •
S. R. Kirnon • P. Palov • V. Polomeno • J. Saroop •
M. Tsang • K. Watson-Jarvis

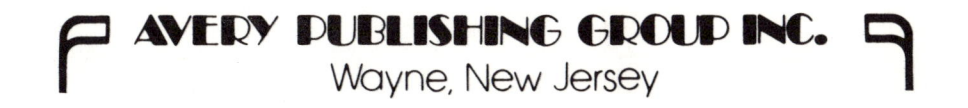

AVERY PUBLISHING GROUP INC.
Wayne, New Jersey

My gratitude and special thanks to my family; my husband John and my girls Belinda and Diane, for the understanding and support they offered me through the preparation of this book.

Cover Photo by Michel Tcherevkoff
Cover Design by Martin Hochberg and Ken Rajman
Text Illustrations by David Rolling
(except for pages 24, 28, 31, by Pamela Tapia)
In-house editors Susan Capasso and Diana Puglisi

Copyright © 1985 by Toula Hatherall

Library of Congress Cataloging-in-Publication Data

Hatherall, Toula, 1944–
   Having babies.

   Bibliography: p.
   Includes index.
   1. Pregnancy. 2. Childbirth. 3. Infants--Care and
hygiene. I. Bresnen, R. II. Title.
RG525.H275   1985   618.2   85–18543
ISBN 0-89529-267-X (pbk.)

All rights reserved. No part of this publication may be reproduced, stored in a retrieval system, or transmitted, in any form or by any means, electronic, mechanical, photocopying, recording, or otherwise, without the prior written permission of the copyright owner.

Printed in the United States of America

10 9 8 7 6 5 4 3 2 1

Contents

Preface   vi
Foreword   viii
To The Reader   ix
Introduction   x

Part I. Pregnancy

1. Roles   3
2. Anatomy and Physiology   6
3. Nutrition for You and Your Baby   12
4. Summary of Monthly Physical, Emotional, and Fetal Changes   24
5. The Expectant Father   27
6. Sexuality During Pregnancy   30
7. Medical Supervision During Pregnancy: Diagnostic Tests and Procedures   32
8. Posture and Back Care   41
9. Prenatal Physical Exercises   44

Part II. Labour and Birth

10. Relaxation   53
11. Labour   57
12. Psychoprophylaxis   66
13. Breathing Techniques for Labour   68
14. Pain—Easing the Way   72
15. Coach's Reminder Sheet   77
16. Guidelines to Couples Participating in Labour   81
17. Induction of Labour and Other Forms of Medical Intervention   88
18. Cesarean Birth   92

Part III. The Postpartum Period

    19. The Postpartum Period   111
    20. Postnatal Exercise Program   117
    21. Breastfeeding   121
    22. Bottle Feeding   130
    23. Infant Care   134
    24. The Grieving Couple   145
    25. Family Planning   147

Bibliography   153
Index   159

Acknowledgements

This book owes a great deal to the childbirth classes that I have been involved with for the last thirteen years. Originating with a collection of materials to cover specific needs, a framework for the development of our childbirth education manual slowly evolved, and eventually led to this book.

I would like to thank my colleagues and co-authors for participating as contributors and making this book possible:

> R. Bresnen P. Palov
> E. Carswell V. Polomeno
> M. Clement J. Saroop
> M. Copp M. Tsang
> B. Gillett K. Watson-Jarvis
> S. R. Kirnon

My heartfelt gratitude goes to Dr. A. Lalonde and Dr. R. Usher for reviewing the entire manuscript and offering suggestions. Additional medical advice was graciously provided by Dr. S. Weeks.

The outstanding artwork is the product of one exceptionally talented young man, David Rolling—my sincere thanks for his assistance.

I would like to thank Cecily Lawson Smith for proofreading the whole manuscript for me in her spare time even though she is a very busy lady.

Acknowledgements are also due to the staff of the physiotherapy department of the Royal Victoria Hospital, the staff dietitians of the Royal Victoria Hospital; "Position Paper on Infant Feeding, P.C.D.Q."; Building Baby, Manitoba Department of Health and Social Development; Dr. J. Stamm, Public Health Dentistry, McGill University.

Last, but not least, I would like to thank my friend Cathy Went for her cooperation and hard work throughout this project.

Preface

While recent advances in perinatalogy, neonatalogy, and genetics have pushed further the frontiers of obstetrics, women have often been left with many questions regarding their pregnancy, the development of their body, and the birthing process. This book offers the prospective father and mother a comprehensive, detailed and well-illustrated outline of modern maternity care.

Compared to many books, this maternity guide has several unique features. The detailed account of anatomy and physiology is complemented by the accurate account in lay terms of the latest developments in perinatal health care: diagnostic tests, hospital procedures, labour, and delivery techniques, including cesarean birth.

This textbook has made inroads in defining and describing the labour coach, this special maternal person who is the basis for a succesful labour and delivery. The father, that often forgotten partner, has a strong role and thus can gain insight into the birthing process.

The chapters on nutrition, sexuality during pregnancy, and cesarean birth, along with the coach's reminder sheet, are innovative, very detailed, and invaluable to expectant couples.

The seven chapters on postpartum care provide the couple with authoritative information on the care of the newborn, family planning, self care and postpartum exercises. A very sensitive text on grieving is another feature of this book.

The references included in this text are exhaustive, and up-to-date, and reflect the author's knowledge of all aspects of the pregnant woman's health care. Her vast experience in the provision of specialized prenatal counselling is surpassed only by her intimate knowledge of the physiology of labour, delivery and postpartum care. Although this book describes the administrative procedures of a large university maternity hospital, it can be easily adapted to any community maternity or birth centre. The author's sensitive treatment of the birthing process makes this book an intimate, frank presentation of the important issues facing parents-to-be. The style is concise and clear, the facts precise, and the scientific concepts are treated in terms that all couples will understand.

The complex nature of conception, fetal development, labour, delivery, and postpartum care is presented with a strong undercurrent of humanity, love, compassion. This textbook belongs to all men and women whose concern for childbirth is only surpassed by their desire for a new beginning.

André-B. Lalonde, m.d. f.r.c.s., f.a.c.o.g.,
f.a.c.s., f.a.b.o.g., c.s.p.q.
Associate Professor, McGill University
Royal Victoria Hospital, Montreal
Chief obs.-gyn.
LaSalle General Hospital

Foreword

Who is best qualified to write a book about having a baby? Professionals who are care givers in the various aspects of the process each possess a great body of knowledge and skill about their particular roles. None can match the breadth of experience of the childbirth educator, however, in dealing with the many-faceted needs and concerns of people from all walks of life who are the aspiring mothers and fathers to be. This book represents the distillation of the experience of one respected nurse-educator whose responsibility it has been to guide many teachers and untold numbers of pregnant learners through the months of preparation for childbearing. It avoids the shoals to lee and to windward, between being too nebulous and too dogmatic, too scientific and too emotional, too sophisticated and too patronizing. In a field where advances and change have been revolutionizing clinical practice, and differences in approach are great from year to year or place to place, there is need for an up-to-date, authoritative, yet not authoritarian, source of information.

The expectant mother and father want practical advice, addressed to specific questions. These chapters will go far to quench the pregnant learners' burning need to know. In dispassionate terms they deal with issues of life and death, sexuality and three-way relationships, and confidence-destroying fears, which are usually found to be baseless.

Just as countless individuals have been helped in person by childbirth educators to try to achieve complete fulfillment of their potential as new parents, this book will reach out to and help many more. It is not an easy task to have a baby; these chapters never let one forget that there is nothing so rewarding. Painful, maybe, fearsome often, worthwhile always.

Robert H. Usher, M.D.
Physician-in-Charge, Neonatology
Associate Professor of Pediatrics,
Obstetrics and Gynecology
McGill University
Montreal, Canada

To The Reader

Although your baby is just as likely to be a girl as a boy, our language, unfortunately, has not provided us with a genderless pronoun. Therefore, to avoid using the awkward "he/she" or the impersonal "it" when referring to the baby, the masculine pronouns "he," "him," and "his" have been used throughout this book. Similarly, we have used the masculine pronouns to refer to doctors and the feminine pronouns to refer to nurses and other health care providers without meaning to imply that this is in any way the preferred situation. These decisions have been made in the interest of simplicity and clarity.

A book of this scope cannot attempt to discuss all of the varied circumstances that may be a part of pregnancy, labour, and delivery. We have focused on situations that occur frequently, but we ask you to bear in mind that we are providing a generalized description, not an account of any particular child's birth.

Introduction

Food, shelter, love, affection, reassurance and the need to reproduce are the primary needs which have been common to all human beings throughout the ages. Methods of meeting these needs may have changed, but the basic family unit remains the same.

For the modern couple, the important prelude to labour and delivery is prenatal education; you need to know what to expect and what will happen in terms which you can understand.

In conjunction with childbirth education classes, this book aims to educate you and to help you evaluate your feelings about pregnancy, thus facilitating an easy adjustment to this new stage in your lives. This concept of care is based on the belief that childbearing and childbirth are natural processes which concern you the family as a unit.

Prepared childbirth is based on the principle that your anxiety can be greatly reduced and your positive feelings reinforced when you become informed about the process of birth; this in turn will enable you to cope more effectively with labour and delivery. Though preparation may not be a complete substitute for drugs and anesthesia, it often reduces the need for them, or reinforces their effects when used.

As you learn breathing and relaxation techniques to use during labour, your partner learns how to coach and comfort you. The cooperation between mother and father fosters a greater understanding and awareness of each other, of the process of birth, and of the responsibility of parenting. Together you will discover that the months ahead can be as rewarding as they are challenging.

You and your partner will learn about the physical and emotional changes during the months of pregnancy as well as about your roles during labour and delivery so that you may both take an active part in these processes.

As well as providing information about the normal events surrounding pregnancy, labour, delivery and infant care, sections have been included on complications, cesarean and grieving. These are not meant to frighten you but rather to inform and strengthen you should the need arise.

As motherhood begins so begins one of the most wonderful experiences in life, an experience which will change you the couple into a family and a man and woman into parents. Both of you emerge with a great sense of joy and satisfaction, because together you have shared a very meaningful experience.

SECTION I:
PREGNANCY

Chapter 1
Roles

The psychoprophylactic preparation for childbirth is a structured program in which all efforts are combined and directed towards Family Centred Maternity Care.

During labour, you and your partner will actively support each other and will aid the professional team in making the delivery (childbirth) a success.

Although this approach can significantly diminish the discomfort of labour, it by no means completely eradicates pain. It is therefore of paramount importance that, as a couple, you are realistic and are motivated to work diligently and patiently throughout labour. Towards this end an effective support system is required. In order that you and your partner complement each other to maximum advantage, you must understand your roles and the roles of the medical and paramedical staff.

The exercises taught by the psychoprophylactic method are based upon the theory of conditioned reflexes. Certain stimuli are introduced in exercise form which override the signals from uterine contractions reaching the brain. By such superimposition, the uterine contractions have less impact and therefore appear less painful. It is important to realize that there are a variety of sensations felt during labour, but *not all* are painful. Hence, there are different ways of coping with these.

Psychoprophylaxis is goal-oriented. Its aim is to provide the most favourable circumstances for the birth of a child and to enable you and your partner to experience as much enjoyment as possible on the threshold of parenthood.

You and your partner must know your individual roles at the outset of labour.

THE PARTURIENT (A WOMAN IN LABOUR)

The role of a woman in labour has greatly changed and expanded. Whereas in the past she played a 'passive" part, she now acts positively, actively and practically to assist the progress of her labour. With psychoprophylactic training and education, you will be conscious of your efforts and your ultimate goal. You will carry out respiratory techniques and other appropriate exercises in a relaxed and rhythmic manner.

You will maintain a good self-image while cooperating as closely as possible with the childbirth team, i.e., partner, doctor and nurse. You will control your own emotional reactions by taking steps to minimize your own discomfort, fear and anxiety. Through conscious effort, you may prevent the need for medical intervention and treatment.

During labour, you will co-ordinate your physical behaviour in response to your uterine contractions and will ultimately obtain satisfaction from determining the success of your own labour.

PARTNER (SUPPORT PERSON)

As a result of psychoprophylactic training, you will be made aware of what your partner will experience during labour. During her pregnancy, you will learn to check her behaviour, attitude and responses so that in labour you will continue to support her emotionally and physically and to monitor her breathing exercises.

Your presence in labour and delivery will provide you with a rich, rewarding experience as a future father. Psychologically, you will be able to overcome your own anxieties by focusing on her performance. You will encourage and reinforce her good efforts and will help her to stay alert. You will learn to be a good friend, coach and, eventually, a parent.

Your commitment and support will be increased as you participate totally in the childbirth experience. Together, you will set your own goals for labour and delivery. You will act as a mediator between your partner and the childbirth team. Your encouragement and support can be an inspiration to her.

Indeed, the experience is profound; if you have done everything possible to help your partner in labour, you will find childbirth an extremely joyful and rewarding experience.

NURSE AS CHILDBIRTH EDUCATOR

The role of the nursing staff is two-fold, encompassing education and care giving. As a childbirth educator, the nurse is responsible for assessing and meeting your needs within the context of the social, cultural, economic, health and emotional factors of your environment. During the course of your childbirth education classes, she will provide you with practical tools such as breathing and relaxation techniques which serve to diminish the discomforts of labour. (In some classes, the breathing and relaxation techniques will be taught by a physiotherapist.) It is also the nurse's duty to discuss with you your goals and expectations of the childbirth experience and to provide knowledge, encouragement and support during your transition to parenthood.

In the role of care-giver, a nurse will be present in the labour and delivery room performing routine nursing functions. At this time, she also has responsibility as an educator. She will be available to explain exactly what is happening and why certain procedures are being used, as well as to provide emotional support and encouragement to you and your partner. During the postpartum period, the nursing staff will help you both learn how to handle the new little person in your lives, they will answer your questions, and will continue to play a supportive role. In short, the nursing staff will cater to both your physical and emotional needs.

OBSTETRICIAN

In order to find the best doctor for you, you must have some notions of what you are looking for. Do you prefer a doctor who encourages you and your partner to ask questions and participate in decision-making? Or a doctor who makes all the decisions? Shop around until you find the doctor that suits your needs.

As well as providing medical supervision during your pregnancy and delivering your baby, it is the obstetrician's responsibility to inform you of possible complications and their treatment. The purpose of this is not to frighten you, but rather to ensure that you are prepared if complications should arise.

You should understand the rationale for and the function of instruments and interventions used during labour. Your doctor should provide an explanation and indications for use of the following: intravenous solutions, induction of labour, artificial rupture of membranes, fetal heart monitor, failure to progress in labour, fetal distress, meconium stained liquor, CPD (cephalo-pelvic disproportion), breech presentation, episiotomy, and forceps. He or she should also explain any side effects of these conditions and/or procedures.

The obstetrician should also discuss with you whether or not your partner will be permitted into the labour and delivery room, or in the case of a cesarean, the operating room. You should be aware of the advantages or disadvantages of your partner's presence, if any, as well as the cooperation which will be required of him.

ANESTHESIOLOGIST

The role of your anesthesiologist is to relieve pain during labour and delivery and to give you an understanding of the cause of pain and how it may best be alleviated. It is his or her responsibility to describe to you the various methods of anesthesia as well as their advantages and disadvantages. He or she should define terms such as: analgesics, tranquillizers, local anesthesia, i.e., paracervical and pudendal blocks, epidural, and general anesthesia.

In the hospitals where the epidural method of anesthesia is most commonly used, you should be fully aware of what to expect. You must be aware of such things as: the rate of effectiveness and duration of action, the position used in labour and in the delivery room, the placement of the epidural catheter and its removal after delivery, and the use of intravenous solutions. You should also be told how you will feel after having had an epidural, and you should be aware of any possible side effects. A discussion as to whether or not your partner may be present during this procedure is also very important.

Ideally, you should meet with the anesthesiologist before your due date so that you can discuss these matters with him or her. However, since this is not always possible, ask questions at your childbirth education classes, ask your doctor, and read as much as you can about the subject.

PEDIATRICIAN

The role of the pediatrician is to help you maintain the health and well-being of your child by following his physical, mental and social growth and development. It is his or her responsibility to advise you about infant care, preventive medicine and the treatment of disease.

He or she will help you deal with common pediatric problems such as: feeding, sleeping, elimination, habits and exercise, etc.; with illness and what signs and symptoms are significant; with nutrition (breastfeeding, bottle feeding, introduction of solids, vitamins and fluoride use, etc.), and with the care of the newborn and infant's skin, eyes, ears, umbilicus, bathing and clothing.

In the realm of preventive medicine, it is the pediatrician's responsibility to meet your child's needs in terms of vaccines, hygiene, accident prevention, poisoning and screen tests, etc. His or her area of specialization is children's medicine and you will find him or her to be a valuable part of a supportive network in your childbearing experience.

Chapter 2
Anatomy and Physiology

During pregnancy, your body will undergo a number of normal anatomical and physiological changes which should be understood in order to render this time of your life a positive and enriching experience. The female reproductive organs may be divided into three categories: internal, external and secondary organs.

1. *Internal Organs*: The internal organs include the uterus or womb, ovaries, fallopian tubes, and vagina.

2. *External Organs*: The external organs include the mons veneris, labia majora and minora, clitoris, and hymen.

3. *Secondary Organs*: The secondary organs include the breasts or mammila.

The reproductive organs play such a major role during pregnancy that they are directly responsible for the bodily changes which appear as pregnancy progresses. The focus, however, will be upon the internal reproductive organs since this is the area in which the most marked and dramatic changes occur.

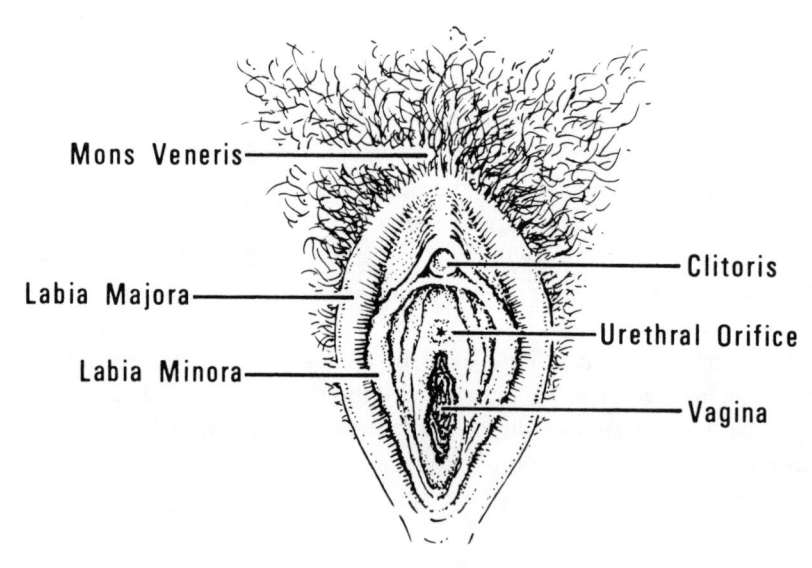

Figure 2.1. External Organs.

THE UTERUS

The uterus is a hollow, thick-walled, muscular organ which lies between the bladder and the rectum and is supported by the broad and round ligaments and by the muscles of the pelvic floor. It is a pear-shaped organ which, due to its muscular make-up, can increase to the size of a basketball. Its bottleneck opening, the cervix, projects into the vagina.

Marked changes occur in the uterus as it makes room for the growing fetus. It can increase from about 6.5 cm long, 4 cm wide, and 2.5 cm deep, to approximately 32 cm long, 24 cm wide, and 22 cm deep. Its weight can increase from 60 gm (2 oz) before pregnancy to as much as 1000 gm (2 lb) at full term.

In its pre-pregnant state, the uterus measures less than one cm in thickness, but during the first few months of pregnancy, its walls can thicken from one to two cm and it has a capacity of two ml. However, as time progresses, the walls decrease in thickness to about 0.5 cm or less, at which time the uterus is capable of containing the fetus, placenta, and over 1000 ml of amniotic fluid. It is the formation of new muscle fibers, the enlargement of the layers of intertwining muscles already present, and the stretching effect of the growing fetus which allows such a stretching of the uterine walls.

The muscles of the pregnant uterus have a greater capacity to contract and, from the first trimester right through to the end of pregnancy, painless uterine contractions occur at intervals of 5 to 10 to 20 minutes. These are called Braxton Hicks contractions. Although you may not be conscious of them at first, you may be able to palpate them in the later months by placing your hands over your abdomen and feeling an alternate hardening and softening of your uterus. The size of the uterus is enlarged by this alternate contraction and relaxation and is thus able to accommodate the growing fetus. It must be noted that these contractions often account for false labour.

THE OVARIES

The ovaries are two almond-shaped organs which are found in the upper part of the pelvis, one on either side of the uterus. They develop the eggs, and then send them out at ovulation. The ovaries are attached to the posterior ends of the broad ligament of the uterus. During pregnancy they are carried up into the abdominal cavity by the enlarging uterus.

The ovaries lie close to the fallopian tubes so that the eggs can easily be picked up at ovulation.

THE FALLOPIAN TUBES

The fallopian tubes extend from the upper and outer sides of the uterus. They are convoluted muscular canals which are very narrow where they enter the uterus. They are lined with hairlike projections which direct the eggs along the tubes into the uterus.

THE VAGINA

The vagina is a canal of muscles and membranes which is connected to the uterus. Bartholin's glands secrete a lubricating substance around the vagina during sexual excitement. Uterine secretions also provide lubrication for the vagina. The vagina has several functions: it is the canal through which the menstrual flow escapes; it is the female organ for sexual union; and it serves as the birth canal during delivery.

In preparation for the passage of the baby at the time of labour, the vagina and external genital organs become thicker, softer, and much richer in blood supply. The increase in blood supply gives a dark violet colour to these tissues, which is in contrast to their usual pink hue. This is a valuable sign of pregnancy and is commonly called "Chadwick's Sign" by your doctor.

Toward the end of your pregnancy, you may notice quite an increase in vaginal secretions. These may be thick, white, and of crumbly consistency. This is a normal occurrence.

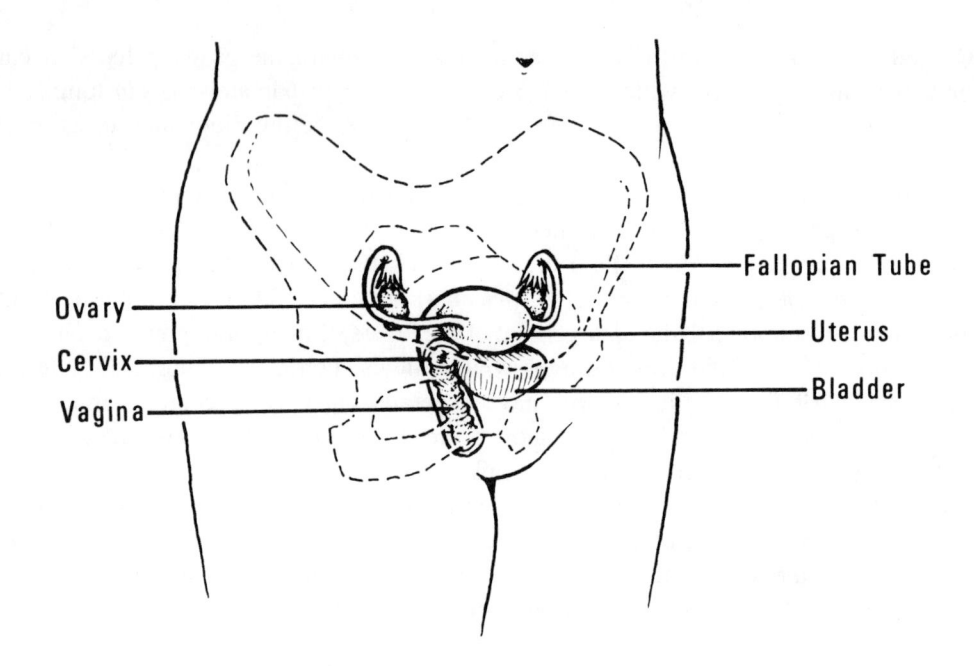

Figure 2.2. Internal Organs.

THE CERVIX

As early as one month following conception, the cervix becomes softer, shorter, larger in diameter, and more elastic. The glands of the cervix, which undergo marked changes and become filled with mucus, almost resemble a honeycomb and make up about half of the entire cervix. This is what is commonly called the "mucus plug" and it is important for various reasons. First, it protects the uterus from contamination by bacteria in the vagina. Its presence also allows for continued activities such as intercourse, swimming and taking a bath. Lastly, the mucus plug along with a small amount of blood are usually the first structures expelled at the onset of labour. This discharge is known as the "show."

THE BREASTS

Changes in your breasts during pregnancy are all directed toward the preparation for breastfeeding. The earliest breast alterations are quite similar to the heaviness and fullness felt prior to menstrual periods, but exaggerated somewhat. In the first few months you may simply feel a tenderness, soreness or tingling of your breasts. It may be after the second month that the breasts begin to become larger, firmer, nodular and more tender. As pregnancy progresses, the nipples and elevated pigmented areas around them (the areola) become darker and wider (from 1½" before pregnancy to 2" to 3" at this time). The tubercles of Montgomery become prominent and, in a few women, patches of brownish discolouration appear on the normal skin surrounding the areola. These patches are called secondary areola and are another sign of pregnancy.

After about the third month, a thin, yellowish fluid can be expressed from the nipples either spontaneously or by massage. This fluid is *colostrum* and precedes the appearance of milk (which does not appear until about the third day after delivery).

An increase in blood supply becomes essential with such an increase in growth and activity of your breasts. Therefore, enlarged blood vessels may be quite prominent during pregnancy as well.

Anatomy and Physiology 9

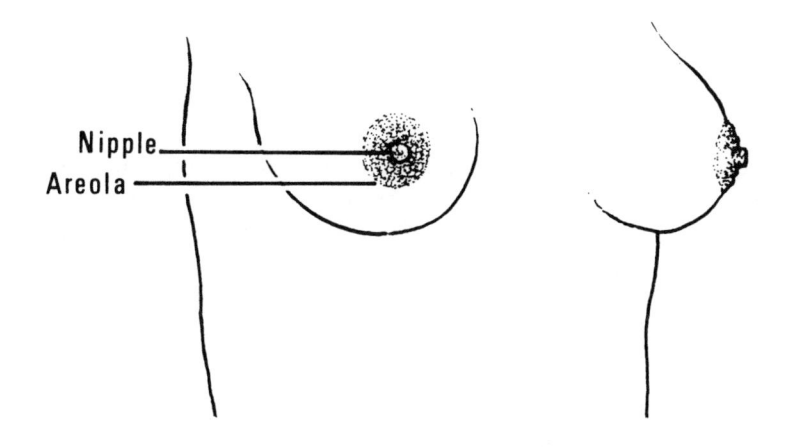

Figure 2.3. Secondary Organs (Breasts).

CHANGES IN OTHER BODY STRUCTURES AND SYSTEMS

Abdomen

As the baby grows and develops and as the uterus extends up into the abdominal cavity, the abdomen naturally becomes larger. The distension of the abdominal wall in the final months of pregnancy sometimes results in certain pink or slightly reddish streaks in the skin covering the sides of the abdomen and upper thighs. They do get lighter after delivery is completed and finally take on a silvery white colour resembling a scar. The number, size, and distribution of these streaks, commonly called *striae gravidarum* or stretch marks, vary in different women.

The umbilicus (or navel), which is deeply indented about the first three months of pregnancy, is continuously being pushed outward with time until approximately the seventh month. At this time its depression is completely invisible. Later it rises above the surrounding area and may project, becoming the size of a walnut. However, it will return to its normal state shortly after delivery.

Cardiovascular System

In order to meet the demands of the enlarged uterus and other bodily changes, there is an increase of approximately 30% of your total volume of blood. This increase in the amount of circulating blood may also be attributed to the excretion of the baby's water through your bloodstream as well as to an increase in salt which would cause water retention.

With such an increase in the amount of circulating blood in your body, your heart has about 50% more blood per minute to pump than it did prior to your pregnancy. This cardiac output follows a pattern, peaking at the end of the second trimester, then declining to the non-pregnant level during the last weeks of pregnancy. This is followed by a sharp rise immediately following delivery.

Swelling of the legs occasionally occurs in the last trimester as a result of blood pooling in the extremities. For mothers who already have varicosities, this can present problems and should be dealt with immediately.

Leg cramps, numbness or tingling during pregnancy may be due to circulatory impairments in your muscles as a result of the pressure exerted by the large and heavy uterus on the veins of your pelvis. Overstretching of the muscles or skin, sluggish drainage of waste materials, as well as the lowering of available calcium in the pregnant mother are other causes of leg cramps. When leg cramps occur during labour they are usually due to hyperventilation.

Respiratory System

Changes in the respiratory system occur as a result of the upward pressure exerted by the underlying enlarging uterus. Some expectant mothers may experience shortness of breath as a result of this, especially in the later months of pregnancy. However, the thoracic cavity, which contains the lungs, does grow sufficiently wide to compensate for the upward pressure of the uterus, and there is actually an increase in the amount of air you can breathe. The increased amount of air is quite essential due to the oxygen demand of both you and your baby's blood.

Metabolic Changes: Weight

Weight gain during pregnancy results from the increase in weight of the contents of the uterus as well as the changes in your metabolism. Other causes of weight gain include water retention, an increase in fatty tissue, and protein storage in your body. The average weight gain during pregnancy is about 9–12½ kg. (or 20 to 28 lbs.). During the first three months you may notice only a small gain if not a slight loss. In fact, about half of this weight is gained in the second trimester and a similar amount in the last trimester.

About 5 kg. (or 11 lbs.) of the weight gained, most of which is fluid, is lost at the time of delivery. Further, though slower, reduction occurs during the next few weeks as a mother's body is returning to its original condition.

MENTAL AND EMOTIONAL CHANGES

Mothers-to-be should not be overly concerned about mental and emotional changes that they can sense within themselves. Some degree of emotional instability as well as mixed feelings about your pregnancy and quick mood changes are characteristic of pregnancy. In fact, even in the ordinary course of events, every influence or circumstance affecting your life, whether it is favourable or unfavourable, will have an effect on your pregnancy and motherhood.

This is not to say that all pregnant women experience nervous manifestations and emotional changes. In fact, the effect of pregnancy on emotions varies greatly. It has been proven, however, that the mental status of a woman who is more unstable emotionally is more likely to be affected by the strain of pregnancy.

THE MALE REPRODUCTIVE ORGANS

It seems that the role played by the male in the creation of a new life is very often underestimated or ignored, while the attention is focused upon the mother's changing body and growing fetus. It is our feeling that the perfection of nature can be better understood and appreciated if the functioning of both partners is properly understood. Thus, we feel it is necessary to include a section devoted to explaining the male reproductive system. This system is made up of the penis, and scrotum, which houses the testicles and a canal system.

The testicles (or testes) are two ovoid bodies which are suspended by the spermatic cord. The spermatozoa (sperm) are produced in the seminiferous tubules of the testicles. At maturity, the sperm are expelled from the testicles toward the seminal vesicles where they unite with the semen and are then ejaculated through the urethra by vigorous pumping of the pelvic muscles. Urine cannot escape at the time of seminal emission.

Anatomy and Physiology 11

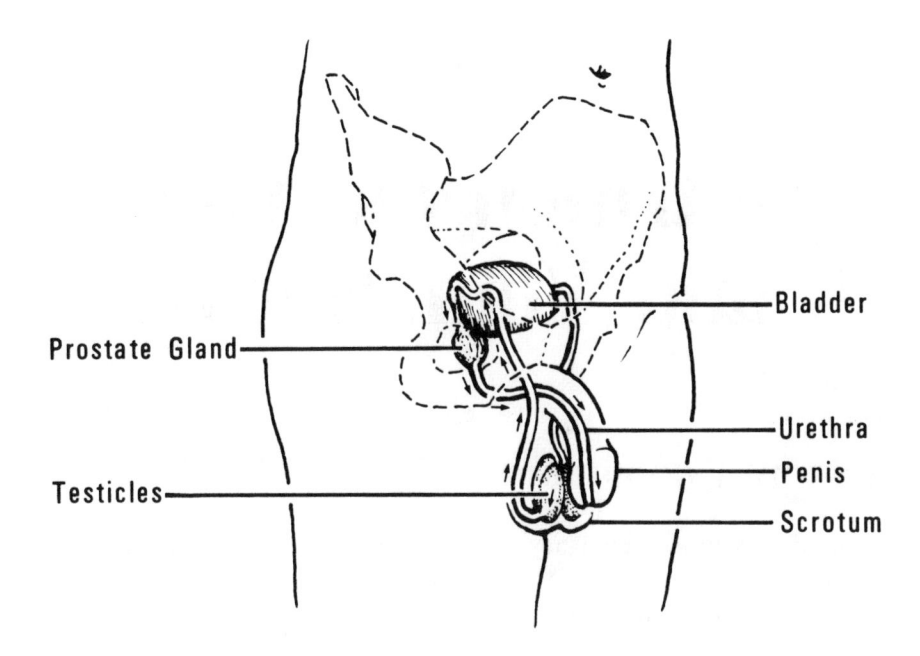

Figure 2.4. Male Reproductive Organs.

It is also interesting to note that it is the male sperm which determines the sex of the child. If there is an X chromosome present, then the child will be female; if the chromosome is Y, then the child will be male.

Chapter 3
Nutrition for You and Your Baby

PREGNANCY—WHY A GOOD DIET?

Good nutrition is important during pregnancy for the proper growth and development of your baby and for your own nutritional well-being. Attention to good dietary habits will help you and your family to develop a better understanding of nutrition and to achieve and maintain better health.

WEIGHT GAIN DURING PREGNANCY

The range of ideal weight gain during pregnancy is 9 to 12.5 kilograms (kg), or 20 to 28 lbs. Women who are underweight will (and should) gain more than will those who are normal or above normal body weight at the beginning of pregnancy.

You can see from the diagram below that this weight is contributed by your growing baby, the placenta, the growth of your own tissues (blood, breasts, uterus, fat stores) and by an increase in tissue fluid late in pregnancy.

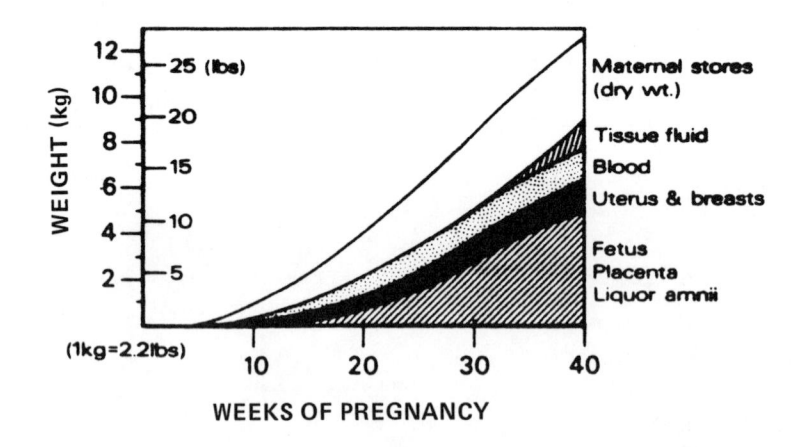

Figure 3.1. The Components of Weight Gain in Normal Pregnancy.
Source: Hytten and Leitch.

The rate of weight gain is even more important than is the total weight gain. During the first trimester (13 weeks) little weight gain occurs, usually 1 to 2 kg (2 to 5 lbs). During the second and third trimesters the rate of weight gain is ⅓ to ½ kg (¾ to 1 lb).

Nutrition for You and Your Baby

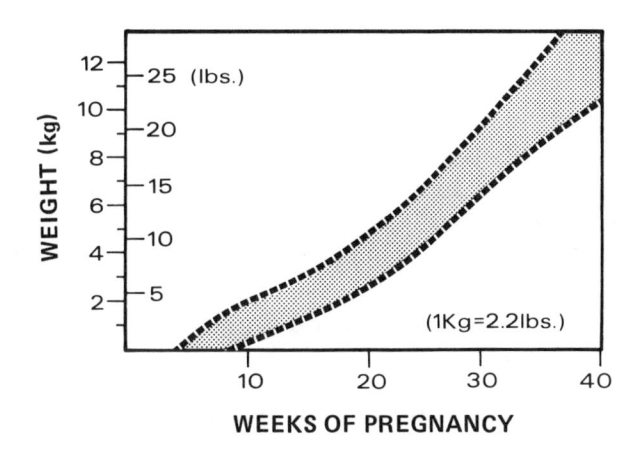

Figure 3.2. Weekly Weight Gain During Pregnancy.

The top line of the graph indicates the pattern of weight gain. The following weight gains are taken from this graph:

        at 10 weeks,   0.65 kg (1½ lb);

        at 20 weeks,   4.0 kg (8¾ lb);

        at 30 weeks,   8.5 kg (18¾ lb);

        and at term,   12.5 kg (27½ lb).

If you have a sudden increase in weight during the last half of pregnancy or if you are not gaining weight at the proper rate, discuss this with your doctor. If you need some help to understand the diagram, discuss it with your doctor or dietitian. At the bottom of this page you will find a chart for recording your weight gain during pregnancy.

    Pregnancy is not the time to lose weight. You need enough energy (calories) to assure a good weight gain. It is important that this energy come from nutritious food. If you are over your ideal body weight, you should consult a dietitian who will help you monitor your weight gain during pregnancy and will help you to revise your energy intake after delivery in order to get back to your ideal body weight. Exercise will help you too.

    If you breastfeed you will need additional food. Weight loss will occur due to milk production. This process is discussed later in this section.

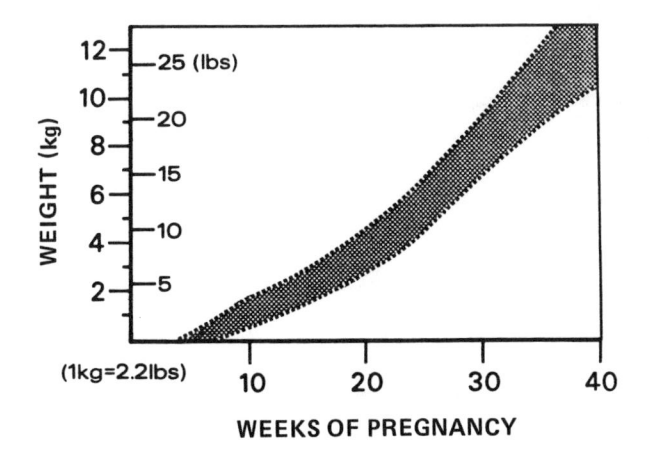

Figure 3.3. Record for Weekly Weight Gain During Pregnancy.
Record your weekly weight gain and compare with the average.

FOOD SELECTION

A guide to help you in food selection follows. Looking at a food guide recommended for use during pregnancy, you can see that your daily food pattern is not very different from Canada's Food Guide. Certain foods are recommended in increased amounts to provide extra vitamins, minerals, protein, and energy which you and your growing baby need.

Your Daily Food Guide

Milk: Drink 4 cups (32 oz or 900mL) of milk daily during pregnancy and 5 cups during lactation.

You need the calcium provided by this milk to provide for bone growth of your baby; otherwise calcium will be drawn from your bones. The extra milk also provides the additional protein needed during pregnancy and lactation.

> If you cannot drink 4 or 5 cups of milk daily, try using part of it in soups, sauces, puddings, casseroles, or drinking it as a milkshake, eggnog, or with Ovaltine. You can also use it on cereal or fruit.
>
> The milk you use may be whole milk (3.5% butterfat); 2% butterfat; or skim milk. The difference is in energy (calories). Whole milk has twice as much energy as skim milk because of the fat content. If you are overweight, the use of a lower fat milk is a good idea.
>
> Skim milk powder is the most economical. Even if you mix reconstituted dried milk half-and-half with whole milk, you can save money.
>
> All milk should have vitamin D added. Low fat milks should have vitamin A added. Read the labels.

Calcium Substitutes for Milk

8 oz (225 mL) milk

    = 1 oz gruyere, parmesan, or swiss cheese

    = 1½ one-inch cubes of cheddar cheese

    = 1½ slices of processed cheese

    = 1 cup yogurt

    = 1 cup milk pudding

    = 1½ cups cottage cheese

    = ½ cup evaporated milk

    = ⅓ cup skim milk powder

Fruit and Vegetables: Three or more servings of fruit, one potato, and three or more servings of other vegetables, preferably dark leafy green or deep dark yellow, and frequently raw.

A serving is one piece of fresh fruit or ½ c. (125 mL) fruit, juice, or cooked vegetable. Good sources of vitamin C (ascorbic acid) are: grapefruit, oranges, tangerines, limes, lemons and their juices; vitaminized apple juice. Other good sources include: tomatoes and their juice, cabbage, salad greens, peppers, cantaloupe, strawberries, broccoli, coleslaw, spinach, and even potatoes. Try to include a second good source of vitamin C daily, either as a fruit or a vegetable.

> Frequent use of raw, dark green, and leafy vegetables will contribute vitamins A and C, folic acid, and iron to your diet. Other nutritious green vegetables include: asparagus, broccoli, Brussels sprouts, cabbage, chard, chicory, endive, kale, leaf lettuce, Lima beans, green beans, okra, peas, peppers, spinach, turnip and beet greens, watercress.

> Examples of deep yellow vegetables are: carrots, pumpkin, sweet potato, yellow squashes. The darker the colour (yellow or green) the more vitamin A contributed to your diet by that vegetable (or fruit).

> Try new vegetables; cook them properly (if you cook them) and eat lots of them. They are low in energy (calories) and high in vitamins and minerals. They also contribute fibre to your diet.

> Remember, vitamin C and folic acid are destroyed by cooking. If you cook vegetables, avoid peeling until after cooking; cook in small amounts of water (or steam or bake) and avoid cutting into small pieces. Cook until just tender, drain, save the cooking water for soup stock, and serve vegetables immediately.

> Always store foods properly (e.g., cover and refrigerate juices once they are opened unless they are to be used right away).

Breads and Cereals: *Five servings* per day. This could be four slices of bread with butter or fortified margarine *plus* one half cup cooked cereal or 1 cup dry enriched cereal per day.

Add one extra serving from this group when breastfeeding. Use whole grain cereals and bread products. They are better because they contribute valuable amounts of fibre to the diet, as well as many other vitamins and minerals.

> Starch food may substitute for some of your bread.

> *Substitutes for One Slice of Bread*

> ½ cup cooked pasta (spaghetti, macaroni, etc.)

> ½ cup cooked rice

> ½ cup cooked cereal or 1 cup dry enriched cereal

> 3 rye crisps

> 4 to 6 whole wheat crackers

Fortified breads, flour, cereals, and pastas, should be used if you purchase refined products. Brown rice is more nutritious than white, but if you use white be sure it is converted (parboiled before milling). Wheat germ adds thiamine, niacin, and some iron to baked products. Oatmeal, millet, whole cornmeal, rye, wheat, and barley cereals are all good. Try to have variety.

Meat, Fish, Poultry, and Alternates: *Four to five ounces* of cooked meat, fish, poultry, or alternates daily.

Protein is necessary for growth and maintenance of your body tissue and that of your growing baby. Every meal and snack should contain some protein.

> *Meat Substitutes*
>
> 2 oz. cooked lean meat, fish, or poultry
>
> 1 cup beans with pork or sausage or weiner
>
> ½ cup cottage cheese
>
> 2 oz. cheese
>
> 2 weiners
>
> 1 medium hamburger patty
>
> 5 link pork sausages (16 per pound)
>
> ⅓ cup canned tuna, salmon, mackerel, or pike
>
> 1 cup cooked dried split peas, lentils, or dried beans
>
> 4 tbsp. peanut butter
>
> 2 meatballs (1-inch diameter) in tomato sauce
>
> 2 eggs
>
> Sardines–one 3¼ oz. tin

If you do not enjoy meat twice a day or if you find it too expensive, the alternates to meat, fish, and poultry listed above will be useful for you.

> For example, try to use a casserole at one meal. Make it with a starch (such as rice, macaroni, spaghetti, etc.) and a good protein source (such as fresh, canned, or frozen fish; dried peas or beans; lentils; nuts; milk; eggs; or cheese).
>
> Less familiar but very nutritious casserole dishes can be made using one of the many varieties of dried peas or beans in combination with brown or enriched rice, buckwheat, or other cereal grains. Stir in a little sharp cheese or cooked bacon or sausage or left-over meat; add onions, celery, mushrooms, spices, and herbs. You will discover interesting, tasty, and nutritious main dishes to serve your family at less cost.

Water: Several glasses daily.

Fluoride: Not important during pregnancy, but it is needed from birth to 16 years of age. Fluoride is incorporated into teeth as they develop and makes them more resistant to decay. Your water supply may be fluoridated; check with your city health department. Then use the table below as your guide for fluoride supplementation. Remember that some commercial infant formula may have fluoride added. Read the label. If you need advice, contact your pediatrician or dentist.

Table 3.1. Recommended Fluoride Supplement

Age	Fluoride Level in Drinking Water		
	.3 p.p.m.	.3 to .7 p.p.m.	.7 p.p.m.
2 weeks to 2 years	0.25 mg/day	0	0
2 to 3 years	0.50 mg/day	.25 mg/day	0
3 to 16 years	1.00 mg/day	.50 mg/day	0

Vitamin D: If you do not consume four or more glasses of milk daily, speak to your doctor about a vitamin D supplement (200 international units per day) or to your dietitian about other sources of vitamin D. This vitamin is needed for the proper utilization of calcium for bone and tooth development.

Iron: Foods rich in iron include liver and other organ meat, meat, and poultry. Also, whole grain breads and cereals and leafy dark green vegetables contain iron. Eat liver once a week. A daily supplement of iron is recommended during the second and third trimesters.

This mineral is needed for building red blood cells to carry oxygen to tissues. The baby needs red blood cells and a storage of iron in his liver for the first few months of life.

Folic Acid: Good sources of folic acid are heart, kidney, liver, leafy green vegetables, dried peas, dried beans, and asparagus. Orange juice, wheat germ, and wheat bran are also good folic acid sources. Because some folic acid is destroyed in cooking, eat your leafy greens raw. Include one of these good sources in your daily diet. If you cannot, you should ask your doctor for a supplement of folic acid. Like iron, folic acid is needed for healthy red blood cells. Inadequate intake of either nutrient can cause anemia.

SUPPLEMENTS

If you consumed a well-balanced diet before pregnancy (including milk, fruits, vegetables, whole grain cereal and bread, and meats or substitutes) and continue this diet throughout pregnancy, there is no need for supplements except for iron and possibly folic acid. Be sure you take your iron supplement every day.

However, if you have not had good eating habits or if you are at greater nutritional risk, you may need other supplements. You should talk to your dietitian and doctor who will decide what your needs are. Remember, taking supplements *does not* substitute for eating nutritious foods.

For example, if you could not tolerate any milk products, a calcium supplement would be given to you. However, milk provides important protein, vitamin D, vitamin A, riboflavin, and some folic acid, as well as other nutrients. Therefore, your total diet should be reviewed when you are omitting an entire food group like this.

SPECIAL NEEDS

Some examples of expectant women who are at greater nutritional or medical risk include those who:

- are under 18 years of age
- are overweight or underweight at the beginning of pregnancy
- have a chronic disease (diabetes, anemia, etc.)
- have poor eating habits for any or several reasons.

All these women fall into a *special group* and all need the personalized help of a dietitian or nutritionist to help plan a diet that will meet special needs. Regular visits to the doctor are also important for these women.

Women who have food habits which do not follow the "traditional" pattern of Canada's Food Guide, for example vegetarians or those belonging to different ethnic groups, should see a dietitian to be sure that they are getting all the required nutrients in sufficient quantities.

ENERGY

Food provides energy for growth during pregnancy and for milk production during breastfeeding. Therefore, the recommended increases above your normal needs are:

- Pregnancy   First trimester, add 100 calories per day
  Second and third trimesters, add 300 calories per day
- Breastfeeding   Add 500 calories per day

If you are gaining weight at the recommended rate, it means that you are eating the right amount. Remember, if you were *underweight* before pregnancy you will and should gain more weight during pregnancy than someone who was of normal body weight before pregnancy.

Where To Get This Energy?

Milk   8 oz. whole milk   150 calories
                           8 oz. skim milk   80 calories

Vegetables   ½ cup cooked vegetable   approx. 35 calories

Fruit   1 serving   approx. 60 calories

Bread   1 slice bread or ½ cup cooked cereal   approx. 70 calories

You can see that by simply adding the recommended 2½ cups of milk (even skim milk) to your daily diet you will, in fact, exceed the recommended increase in calories for the first trimester. Actually you do not need to count calories every day. The important thing is to follow the Food Guide and avoid taking calories from foods that are not nutritious. Take a good look at your present diet. It may need some changes.

How Should You "Revise" Your Diet?

An easy way is to compare your usual daily intake to the Daily Food Guide for pregnancy (which appears on page 20). Do you get the recommended number of servings of each food group? You will notice that common desserts and snack foods are not listed. When selecting snacks and desserts, you should choose from the food groups too!

One of the best ways to improve the quality of your diet and to limit excess calories is to restrict your intake of high-calorie desserts and snacks and to eliminate "empty calorie" foods. Examples of "empty calories" are sugars (table sugar, jams, jellies, honey, candies, syrups, soft drinks, etc.) and cooking oils. These make no (or little) contribution to your daily vitamin and mineral intake, but may add a considerable number of calories.

It takes motivation and discipline, but it can be done! Replace these nutrient-poor foods with foods from the food groups. The quality of your diet, your growing baby's diet, and your family's diet will be better. A guide for some sample menus appears on the next page. The page following will show you the approximate number of calories in the different food groups.

SNACKING

You may find you are hungry between meals. Between-meal appetite can be satisfied by keeping some of your regular meal for later consumption. For example, save your fruit and milk until an hour or two after your meal.

If you want to add extra to your daily food intake, choose fresh or unsweetened fruits, vegetables, skim milk, skim milk cheese or cottage cheese, and whole wheat or enriched crackers or bread, plain yogurt, a few peanuts (they contain protein, but are high in energy). These snacks will satisfy you and will contribute important nutrients to your daily intake in relationship to the energy (calories) they contain. Snacks should be as nutritious as your meals.

Avoid These or Use Them Sparingly

- sugars, soft drinks, and sweetened beverages
- pastries, cakes, pies, candies, chocolates, doughnuts, and all such sweets
- pretzels, chips, and all snack-type crackers and nibblers
- fried foods (keep them to a minimum)
- cream, extra margarine and butter, excessive use of nuts
- beer, alcohol, wine (they are nutrient poor)

SALT

There is no need to restrict salt during pregnancy except for a medical reason. Try adding flavour with herbs and spices in addition to normal use of iodized salt.

CAFFEINE

Caffeine is a drug too, a stimulant which should be avoided during pregnancy. If not totally cut out of your diet, your intake of caffeine should be limited to two to three cups of coffee or tea per day.

Drinking 'café au lait' will stretch your coffee further and help get your milk in. Try cereal beverages (e.g., Postum, Ovaltine) and decaffeinated beverages in moderation. When thirsty you should drink milk, juice, or water in preference to coffee and tea.

Table 3.2. Daily Menu Samples Based on Canada's Food Guide

Breakfast

½ cup orange juice or ½ grapefruit
or ½ cup vitaminized apple juice
½ cup to ¾ cup cereal
½ cup milk

Mid Morning

4 wheat crackers or 1 slice toast, buttered
1 slice processed cheese or 1 inch cube cheddar cheese
½ cup milk

Lunch

1 cup chili con carne
or 1 cup spaghetti with two meatballs
1 slice whole grain bread with butter
coleslaw or tomato sliced with lettuce
1 peach or pear or orange
½ cup of milk

Mid Afternoon

1 cup yogurt or milk
1 canned peach half or small banana

Supper

3 oz. of poultry or fish or meat
½ cup broccoli or baked squash or carrots
1 cup spinach and mushroom salad
1 medium potato
½ cup custard or milk pudding

Evening

1 slice buttered toast or 4 whole wheat crackers
or ¾ cup enriched dry cereal
1 cup milk

Table 3.3. Food Groups and Daily Caloric Intakes

Food Group	Average Serving Size	Number of Servings Per Day	Average Calories Per Serving	Total Calories From Food Group
Milk, whole	250 mL	4	150 Cal.	600 Cal.
Fruit	1 piece or 125 mL	3	60 Cal.	180 Cal.
Vegetables				
cooked	125 mL	3	35 Cal.	105 Cal.
salad	250 mL	1	35 Cal.	35 Cal.
Bread/Cereal	1 slice	5	70 Cal.	350 Cal.
Meat & Substitute	60–75 g 125 mL legumes	120–150 g total 1	160–200 Cal. 100 Cal.	400 Cal. 100 Cal.
Butter, Oil or Margarine	30 mL	30 mL total		250 Cal.
Miscellaneous	Salad dressing or sauce			approx. 100 Cal.
			Approximate Daily Total	approx. 2,100 Cal

ALCOHOL

When you drink an amount of alcohol that is greater than the amount your liver can metabolize, the alcohol passes into your blood supply that goes to the placenta and then passes into the baby's blood. Thus you must never consume any large amount at one time. It is recommended that you completely avoid alcohol throughout your pregnancy. However, if you do drink, limit liquor to one ounce, wine to three ounces, or beer to eight ounces on any single day and only drink on occasion. Always eat, even just a snack, when you drink and sip your drink slowly so that the absorption of alcohol is delayed. This allows your liver time to metabolize the alcohol as it arrives in the liver and it therefore does not spill over into the blood that circulates to the baby.

MEDICINES AND DRUGS

Never take any medications, drugs, or household remedies without consulting your doctor. Most drugs can pass the placenta and may harm your baby.

SMOKING

Statistics show that women who smoke have smaller babies. Smoking causes constriction of blood vessels, including those which supply the placenta. It appears that the result is a reduction in the nutrient supply to the fetus. Smoking also doubles the risk of prematurity and of intrauterine growth retardation, and significantly increases the risk of perinatal death. However, smoking is the major health hazard faced by the fetus that you can do something about. Women who smoke can reduce the risk to their baby by reducing or stopping their smoking while they are pregnant. It is recommended that you not smoke during pregnancy or breastfeeding.

EXERCISE

All kinds of moderate exercise are good for you and should be continued during pregnancy. Swimming, golf, dancing, walking, hiking, tennis, badminton, etc., can be continued. However, don't undertake a vigorous new sport just now. Whatever you are doing avoid tiring yourself, and be sure to get plenty of rest.

A FEW MINOR PROBLEMS

Nausea and Vomiting

Severe "morning sickness" is not very common. The majority of women experience occasional nausea and possibly vomiting which may occur at any time of the day. It should not occur after three months of pregnancy.

If you feel nauseated in the morning, it frequently can be relieved by eating a few dry crackers before getting up. It is best to keep something in your stomach throughout the day and not to go for long periods without food. Try distributing your food into smaller, more-frequent meals. You may find it helpful to take fluids an hour or so after solid foods. Many women find that nausea is best controlled by regular meals and plenty of rest.

If you have persistent morning sickness, you should inform your doctor. He or she may be able to help you through this period of time with a medication. Be sure to discuss this problem with your dietitian too. He or she may be able to help you by suggesting a few changes in your eating habits.

Constipation

Constipation is very common during pregnancy, especially during the last trimester, and this is in part due to the normal changes that take place in your body. Your smooth muscles are more relaxed. The muscles of the digestive tract are mainly smooth muscles.

To avoid constipation you should eat plenty of fibre, drink plenty of water, and exercise daily. Fibre is found in whole grain cereals and breads, and in fruits and vegetables, especially when eaten raw. You can add extra fibre by using a little bran daily on cereals or in cooking.

Try to develop and maintain regular bowel habits. After breakfast is a good time for a bowel movement as the ingestion of fluids and food on an empty stomach stimulates the digestive tract. Many people find a glass of warm water, perhaps with a little lemon juice before breakfast, is an effective way to stimulate a bowel movement. Never use mineral oil or laxatives. If you continue to have constipation talk to your doctor.

Indigestion

Indigestion, heartburn, and gas are common complaints and tend to be more frequent as pregnancy progresses. This is because the growing baby presses up against the stomach and also because smooth muscles are relaxed. Do not treat indigestion with soda and antacids; see your doctor. Avoid foods which tend to cause discomfort, but be sure to replace them with substitutes from their food group if they are nutritious foods. Distribute your food into smaller, more frequent meals. This will decrease the volume of food in your stomach at any one time. Try to take fluids before or after solid foods.

BREASTFEEDING

Will You Breastfeed?

Whether or not to breastfeed is something only you can decide and you should make this decision early during pregnancy. Discussions with your doctor and your husband will help you make the best decision for you and your baby.

Human milk is produced especially for human babies and so is the best food for the baby's nutritional needs. It is more easily digested and it allows certain nutrients such as iron and protein to be more easily absorbed into the blood stream. Infections of the intestinal tract are seen less frequently in breastfed infants because human milk provides an immunity to such infections. Also, fewer allergies are seen in breastfed babies.

A baby can control the amount of milk taken more easily if breastfed. In addition, the composition of breast milk changes slightly during a feeding and this is believed to trigger the satisfaction of appetite. Both these factors help prevent overfeeding the babies.

Milk production requires energy, and the calories you stored during pregnancy will be used up to help perform this work. Therefore, it may help you to return to your ideal body weight.

Finally, breastfeeding is the most economical way to feed your baby.

Breastfeeding is not the only alternative, however. If you plan to bottle feed, use commercial formulas designed to be like mother's milk. Compare products and prices, and talk to your doctor, dietitian, or nurse.

If you decide to breastfeed your baby, you must continue to eat according to the basic food pattern followed during pregnancy (see page 20). Add an extra cup of milk or its equivalent, at least one serving of fruit which is a good source of ascorbic acid, and extra vegetables, other fruits, and one more serving of whole grain cereal or bread.

The energy cost of producing milk is considerable. This extra energy comes from two sources: from the extra food you eat and from the energy reserve which you stored during pregnancy. For each 100 calories used by your body to produce milk, about 80 calories worth of milk are produced. The rest of the energy is used to make the milk.

Protein intake is important too. Your five cups of milk will contribute significantly to your protein intake. Be sure to take a good source of protein at each of your three meals, and try to use snacks that have some protein, such as nuts, peanut butter, or cheese with whole wheat bread or crackers, milk drinks, yogurt, milk puddings, fruits, etc. Good protein sources need not be expensive. Try casserole dishes with cheaper cuts of meat, or fish, or eggs and cheese, or beans with grains such as rice.

A good fluid intake is necessary. In addition to your milk, drink fruit juices and water. You need to replace the fluid lost in your milk and avoid constipation.

As in pregnancy, you may find that some foods are not well tolerated. Try and substitute these with similar foods from the same food group. In most cases these are not important foods. In fact, they tend to be spices, pickles, garlic, and chocolate, all of which are nutritionally unimportant.

APPROXIMATE METRIC MEASURES TO HELP YOU CONVERT WEIGHTS AND VOLUMES

250	millilitres	=	1 cup (8 oz.) volume
30	millilitres	=	1 oz. volume
110	grams	=	½ cup (solids) weight
30	grams	=	1 oz. weight
1	kilogram	=	2.2 pounds

INFORMATION AND RESOURCES

There are courses and counselling available for pregnant women and their husbands. Call your local hospital, health department, or community clinic. The Canadian Government's Health Promotion branches also have information. There are many dietitians offering private consultations. A list of names is available from the office of your provincial dietetic association.

Chapter 4
Summary of Monthly Physical, Emotional, and Fetal Changes

The expectant mother will experience a number of physical and emotional changes during the nine months of her pregnancy. This chapter summarizes these changes in tabular form. Of course, every pregnancy is unique, so your experience may differ from the descriptions given here. This chapter also includes a month-by-month summary of the various changes that take place as the fetus grows and develops, providing an "overall view" of the different stages of pregnancy. The illustration below shows fetal development throughout pregnancy.

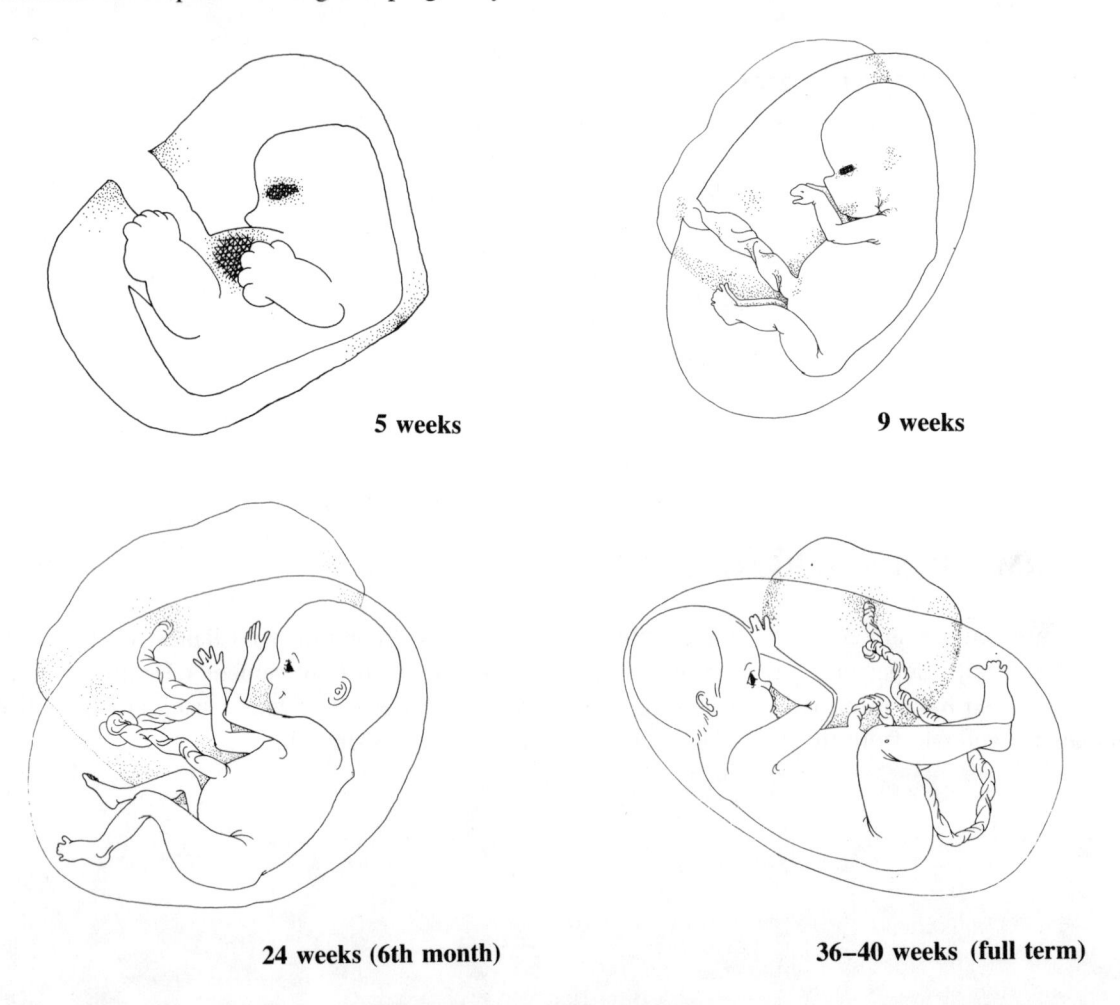

5 weeks

9 weeks

24 weeks (6th month)

36–40 weeks (full term)

Figure 4.1. Fetal Development.

Summary of Monthly Changes

Table 4.1. Summary of Changes.

Physical Changes	Emotional Changes	Fetal Changes
First Month • Ovulation with fertilization • Implantation of fertilized ovum • Thickening of the uterine lining as a result of increased estrogen and progesterone levels • Temperature rises and remains up • Nausea and vomiting • Breasts tingle • Fatigue • Menstruation ceases (some women continue to have light periods for two or three months)		*First Month* • Cell differentiation
Second Month • Positive pregnancy test • Pressure on bladder with frequency of urination • Nausea subsides • Profuse, thick vaginal discharge • Breasts larger • Montgomery's glands may appear on areola • Mucous plug forming in cervical canal	*First Trimester* The following are common feelings during the first trimester: • Ambivalent feelings towards the pregnancy • Excitement about the new life growing within • Increased creativity • Increased sensuality • Extreme mood swings	*Second Month* • Head (largest part), brain, and nervous system forming • Heart developing and starting to beat • Circulation begins • Placenta taking shape • Facial features, arms, hands, fingers, legs, feet, and toes forming • Eyelids begin to form • Nose short and snub • Ears start to take shape
Third Month • Placenta completely formed and is secreting estrogen and progesterone • Uterine cavity filled • Uterus rising from pelvic cavity into abdomen • Colostrum may be expressed from breasts • Nausea subsides • Bladder pressure less • Gums may soften • Thyroid gland may be more prominent		*Third Month* • About 10 cm. or 4 in. long • Human appearance • All organs formed • Sex distinguishable

Table 4.1.—*Continued.*

Physical Changes	Emotional Changes	Fetal Changes
Fourth Month • Visible signs of pregnancy (clothes must be worn looser for comfort) • Quickening (movement of baby is felt) • Blood volume starts to increase • Linea nigra (a dark vertical line on abdomen) may appear	*Second Trimester* The following are common feelings during the second trimester: • Mounting excitement as baby moves and becomes a reality • You may feel special as the pregnancy becomes obvious and you become the centre of attention in your family and in groups of friends • Fears are sometimes brought to consciousness in the form of dreams	*Fourth Month* • Hair forming on head • Lanugo (downy hair all over body) appears • About 16 cm. long
Fifth Month • Placenta covers half of uterine wall • Umbilicus may pop out and remain that way until after delivery • Relaxation of smooth muscles		*Fifth Month* • Vernix (protective coating) forming on skin • Fetal heartbeat may be heard through a stethoscope • Eyebrows and lashes formed • About 25 cm. long
Sixth Month • Greatest weight gain starts • Striae (stretch marks) may appear on abdomen, thighs, or breasts • Chloasma (mask of pregnancy) may appear • May experience heartburn		*Sixth Month* • Outline of baby can be felt abdominally • Skin red and shiny • Face wrinkled • Old man appearance • About 32 cm. long
Seventh Month • Braxton-Hicks contractions palpable • Blood volume highest	*Third Trimester* The following are common feelings during the third trimester: • A great deal of attention focused on the baby, labour and delivery • The baby is perceived as a real person, separate from you • Sometimes self-image becomes negative because of large size	*Seventh Month* • Period of most rapid growth • Viable (capable of life outside the uterus) • Eyes open
Eighth Month • Braxton-Hicks contractions stronger • Striae more pronounced • Backache		*Eighth Month* • Body rounding out • If born, good chance of survival • Head down position • About 44 cm. long • About 2.5 kg
Ninth Month • Shortness of breath • Varicosities • Ankle swelling • Lightening (baby drops) easier breathing • Urinary frequency		*Ninth Month* • Body well rounded • Lanugo shed • About 55 cm. long

Chapter 5
The Expectant Father

During the last few years, the male attitude towards pregnancy and labour has undergone a dramatic change. In the past, it seemed that the father's tasks were simply the act of impregnation and providing a sexual role model for children. Now, however, he is called upon to be actively involved from the beginning of the pregnancy and throughout the childbearing years as a supportive, understanding, and enthusiastic partner. He too can share in the adventure of pregnancy and labour and can witness the wonder of the birth of his own child.

The advantages of maintaining an intact family unit cannot be emphasized enough. As well as promoting bonding, the early establishment of a relationship between parent and child, it also permits the father to participate in the total responsibility for childbearing. Thus, your partner's later parenting may be enhanced if he can become actively involved in the acknowledgement, acceptance, and expression of emotions which pregnancy elicits.

During pregnancy your body goes through a number of changes which make you emotional and irritable, yet you are well equipped to meet the increased demands of your condition. For your partner, however, there are no physical changes brought about by pregnancy, and it is unlikely that he will seek assistance in dealing with whatever physical and emotional stresses pregnancy may induce. He is expected to provide you with emotional support, but his own needs are usually neglected. His transition to parenthood is less smooth than is yours because he undergoes none of the physiological changes which reinforce the reality of the baby.

Your partner's experience of the pregnancy will seem to be very different from yours. All his information is secondhand; even the doctor knows about the pregnancy before he does. He may be surprised and have mixed feelings about news of the pregnancy even if it was planned. He may feel a flash of pride in his virility, but this can often give way to guilt feelings for "getting you pregnant," especially when he sees you struggling with morning sickness or fatigue.

While you may become introverted during the first trimester, your partner might feel left out and neglected. This could cause him to become jealous of the baby and the doctor who have suddenly become such an important part of your life. He may become insecure about his competence as a man and a provider. At this time when he needs a little love and close physical contact, you may be uninterested and not able to provide what he needs.

At this point, it is important that feelings are communicated in order that the gap which separates the two unique experiences of the pregnancy is not widened.

During the second trimester, your partner will be able to experience the reality of the baby when he sees the obvious physical changes in your body and when he is able to feel the movement of the baby. If he still has mixed feelings about the pregnancy, then your physical changes may serve to intensify them. It is imperative that these feelings are expressed and dealt with. You can often assist by expressing strong dependency needs and increasingly seeking the presence and support of your man, thus letting him know that he is indispensable to the family unit.

By the beginning of the third trimester, both of you will begin to emerge from your separate emotional worlds and it is hoped that your partner will have worked through at least some of his emotions surrounding the pregnancy.

At this point, it is easier to focus on physical preparations for the baby, and your partner will spend a great deal of his time fantasizing about his future relationship with you and the child.

If he has anxiety regarding labour and delivery, it might be a problem for him, since he may be afraid to place this burden on you thus violating his role as protector. If he has decided to be present at the birth, he may be worried about how he will react and whether or not he can take it.

And yet, his presence during labour is of utmost importance since he is at the centre of the drama by your side. It is he who will rub your back during the first stage; he who will regulate and correct your breathing and see that you are fully awake and concentrating in your task. It is your partner who will help you to check that you are relaxed; and it is against him that you will lean as you give birth to your child. Perhaps he will be the first person to see the baby. This is the place where your partner belongs. It is not only ludicrous but also pathetic to leave him sitting nervously in a waiting room while you experience the wonder of a new life surrounded by strangers.

Reassurance, active assistance, and loving care from your partner should not be denied since he is, after all, the father of this child who is making its way into the world. Your partner can and should be the one person you feel you must have with you. He should be with you to share the first beautiful and awesome moments of parenthood, rather than being informed, after the fact by a stranger, that he is the father of a son or daughter.

J. Hines states it beautifully: "The price paid for asepsis has often been the blocking of early developmental ties at a time when new families need help most in getting themselves established."[1]

It is a good idea for you and your partner to see the maternity unit before the baby is due, to familiarize yourselves with this new environment and to see any equipment which may be used during labour. When equipment must be used, some men feel that they are no longer needed because the

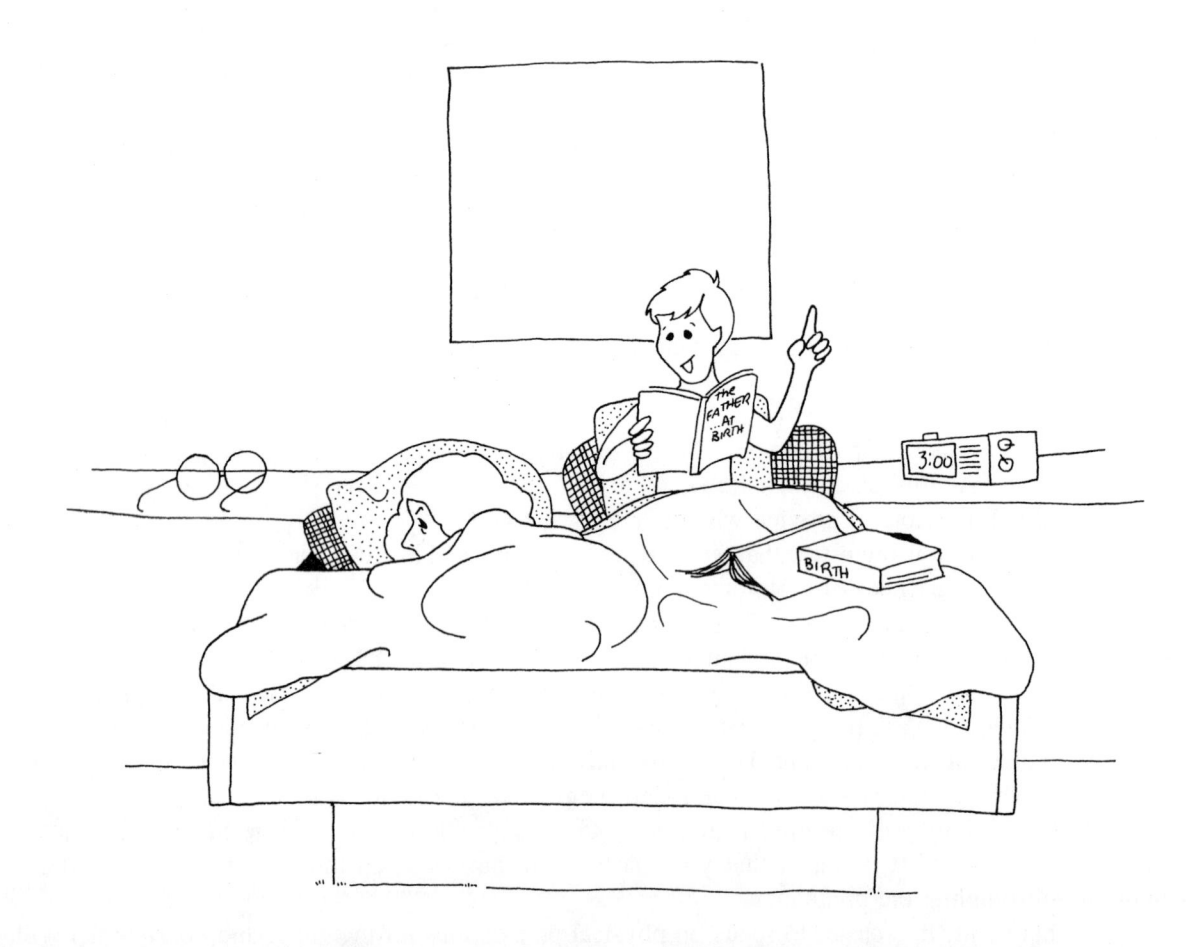

"You know, this isn't going to be as hard as I thought."

machine has taken over; but there is no reason why your partner should not continue to offer loving support and encouragement. The right place for your husband is still by your side. It can be very frustrating for a father to be removed during an emergency, after he has gone through all the preparations for a partner-coached birth. However, if your partner's presence is not possible, you should both try not to feel a sense of failure.

Paternal involvement in postpartum activities may facilitate an early affectional bond formation. M. Greenberg stated that the period within the first three hospital days was critical to the formation of this affectional bond system.[2]

It has been found that visual contact was crucial to initial maternal-infant bonding. While its value in paternal infant bonding is not to be diminished, visual cues alone are not enough to meet the need of the father. Touch or physical contact is one of man's most powerful modes of communication. The need for it begins at birth and continues throughout our life span. For this reaosn it is important that it be incorporated into the early interaction within the father-infant dyad.

Research has demonstrated that the mother's participation in immediate postpartum activities facilitated the all-important mother-infant bonding. These activities include cuddling, touching, inspecting, gazing, and singing. In view of these findings, it would seem that the father's participation in similar activities would also be necessary for a successful bonding relationship.

If the family is to be viewed as a unit, then your partner must be actively involved throughout the pregnancy. This should include open communication between you regarding your fears and fantasies, thus aiding you to consolidate your personal strengths and more fully meet each other's needs.

It is also important that your partner be included immediately following the birth so that he too may participate in the bonding process. If, however, he is not included in early bonding during the hospital stay, then he will be less easily integrated into the family unit.

We cannot emphasize enough that love, mutual consideration, and understanding are the key elements necessary in the transition to parenthood. You and your partner can help each other become the kind of parents you want to be; a father and a mother sharing the responsibility and the joy.

FOOTNOTES

[1] Hines, J. "Father, the Forgotten Man," *Nursing Forum* 10: 177–200, 1971.
[2] Greenberg, M., and Monis, N. "Engrossment: The Newborn's Impact Upon the Father," *AMJ Orthopsychiatry* 44: 520–531, 1974.

Chapter 6
Sexuality During Pregnancy

Pregnancy, with its promise of a new family member, is a beautiful and exciting major event which is bound to bring a radically changing self-image for the expectant mother. She will often wonder about the desirability of her changing body and will question her ability to cope with the dual roles of wife and mother.

This struggle may occur at either the conscious or subconscious level and the woman experiencing it will often grow introspective and withdraw from those who are closest to her. Thus, while she may crave tenderness and reassurance from her partner, she may not be particularly interested in sexual stimulation or intercourse.

It should be noted that there are also a number of physical factors which may influence the pregnant woman's interest in sexual activity. During the first trimester she may experience great fatigue, nausea, vomiting, and enlarged breasts which cause soreness and nipple tenderness. Her sense of touch is heightened, causing her to be sometimes irritated and sometimes sexually stimulated when caressed. Also, there may be an increase in vaginal discharge which is different in odour from the pre-pregnant discharge, and may therefore be offensive to one or both partners.

Many couples wonder if they should have intercourse at all for fear of causing bleeding, miscarriage, or harm to the baby. For this reason the following discussion should answer any questions you may have and set your fears to rest.

Bleeding on penetration is often due to the rupture of small vaginal blood vessels. During pregnancy, the integrity of the walls of superficial blood vessels is threatened and slight bleeding on intercourse or after vaginal examination is not unusual. Shallow penetration will often alleviate bleeding and will feel more comfortable. However, if you feel anxious about the bleeding or if it is accompanied by low abdominal or back pain, call your doctor.

If you have had several miscarriages, you should consider abstaining from sexual stimulation or intercourse during the time at which your menstrual period would normally occur. This is advisable for the first trimester and for the six weeks prior to your due date.

Oxytocin is a hormone which circulates through your body when the breasts and nipples are stimulated and upon orgasm. Interestingly, it is the same hormone which initiates labour. Because of the effects of oxytocin, you may experience rhythmic contractions following sexual activity. This is normal and as the hormonal blood level decreases, so too will the contractions. While the oxytocin level does not rise sufficiently during orgasm to initiate labour, if your cervix is ripe and your body ready, then sexual stimulation will encourage the initiation of the first stage. Once you are in labour, sexual stimulation will speed up the process.

Many women sense a certain discomfort at the pelvic floor and the perineum. This is partially due to the pressure of the uterus against the pelvic floor. During pregnancy, a woman's blood volume increases 25% to 30% and results in vaginal congestion. Because of this condition, your partner may feel that there will not be enough room for his penis. However, with proper foreplay, the vagina will balloon, forming a tentlike structure which is large enough to receive the erect penis.

Due to perineal congestion, the pregnant woman is in a pre-stimulated state and will therefore require less stimulation to achieve orgasm. Also, many women who have never experienced orgasm will do so during gestation. Some women become multi-orgasmic.

Sexuality During Pregnancy

The baby is well protected in the uterus and there should therefore be little fear of hurting him during intercourse. The penis does not reach him and he is floating in the "bag of water" which acts as a shock absorber. Also, the mucus plug in the cervix, or entrance to the uterus, protects him from germs or foreign material.

Some people feel that the baby may be watching or listening to their sexual activity. He cannot see; and although sound waves do reach him, having no past experience, it would be somewhat difficult for him to make any kind of association.

The only caution during pregnancy (or at any other time) is to avoid "blowing" into the vagina, as an air bubble or embolism may reach the circulation of mother or baby. This could be fatal.

During the second trimester, many women feel more comfortable and sensuous and are able to engage in normal sexual activity. For some, the activity is even more enjoyable than before pregnancy because they are free from the effects of contraception and perhaps because they are drawn closer to their partners in the shared, happy anticipation of the new life growing within.

By the sixth month of pregnancy, some couples realize that previous sexual positions are no longer attainable. Thus, it is important that the matter be discussed openly and that alternatives which are acceptable and pleasurable to both partners can be discovered.

It may mean that caressing and massaging of the clitoris or penis becomes an option. Oral sex, if conducted gently, may also be quite pleasurable and acceptable. You may find that entry from the rear or side position is more comfortable, as the weight of your partner is not pressing down upon your abdomen. This can easily be executed in a lying, kneeling, or standing position. If one partner lies on his/her back while the other faces and kneels, entry can be very accessible and penetration will not be too deep.

Pregnancy is an excellent time for you and your partner to abandon old routines and to embark upon an exciting voyage of sensuous discovery.

Following the delivery of the baby, intercourse should not be resumed until the lochia becomes brown or pinkish.

The first intercourse after the delivery may be painful, so spend an early evening together, relax and take your time. If you are breastfeeding, feed the baby just prior to making love. In this way your breasts will be empty and will not leak and the baby will be full and will not interrupt.

It may take a while to resume a regular routine. Vaginal lubrication is scarce until your first period so that a jelly may be necessary to facilitate entry.

It will take time to become accustomed to the sounds of the new baby and to relax and not feel that he is needing you. Sometimes you and your partner will be too tired to do anything but hold each other.

Talk things over, take your time, and enjoy.

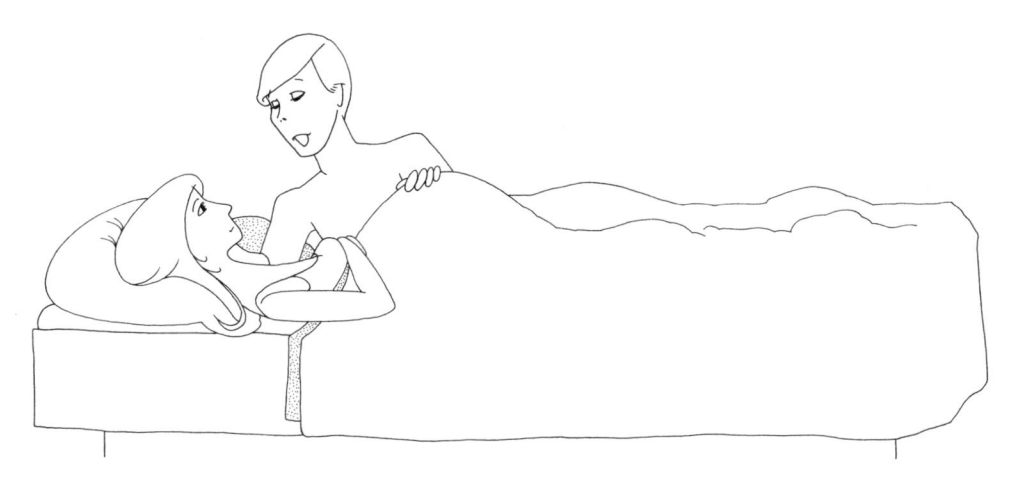

"Well . . . at least we can still be friends."

Chapter 7

Medical Supervision During Pregnancy: Diagnostic Tests and Procedures

Ideally, all couples should have a thorough medical examination complete with detailed personal and family history prior to conception. The information collected would reveal possible problem areas affecting the outcome of the pregnancy such as: blood incompatibilities, infections, genetic disorders, alcohol or drug problems, nutritional deficiencies, etc. Informed couples would be better prepared to produce healthy children.

Since most couples are not yet oriented towards the ideal preventative medical approach to childbearing, the medical detective work is often done during the pregnancy.

It is advisable for the pregnant woman to see her doctor as early as possible during pregnancy and regularly thereafter. The exam schedule usually includes monthly visits to the doctor until the eighth month, visits every two weeks during the eighth month, and weekly during the ninth month until birth. A postpartum visit is scheduled approximately six weeks after the birth.

Group practice in obstetrics is convenient for the medical team but disconcerting to many patients. The expectant mother establishes a rapport with her doctor during the prenatal period only to be delivered by a complete stranger: another member of the "group" who happens to be on duty that day. Some obstetrical groups are attempting to overcome this problem by scheduling their patients' regular prenatal visits with other members of the team. This way the expectant mother, while being followed primarily by her own doctor, gets to meet each of the other doctors in the group at least once.

THE ROUTINE OBSTETRICAL CARE WILL LIKELY INCLUDE[1]

1. *Medical History:* menstrual history, previous pregnancies, operations, illnesses (e.g., German measles—rubella), drugs taken, history of family illnesses such as heart disease, kidney disease, diabetes, anemia.

2. *General Physical Exam*

3. *Exam for Pregnancy* including:

    a. Examination of *breasts* to see if there are any changes in the glands. Later in the pregnancy the *nipples* should be checked to rule out the possibility of flat or inverted nipples, which could interfere with breastfeeding. Inverted or flattened nipples can be treated prenatally by nipple preparation techniques and possibly by different shields.

Medical Supervision/Diagnostic Tests 33

    b. *Pelvic examination* (internal) which shows the position and consistency of the uterus, condition of the ovaries and fallopian tubes, consistency and colour of the cervix.
    c. *Pap test, vaginal smear and culture*
    d. *Blood tests for*
       blood group
       Rh factor
       complete blood count
       hemoglobin
       hematocrit (device for separating the cells and other particulate elements of the blood from the plasma)
       sugar
       syphilis
    e. *Complete urinalysis* and regular testing of the urine for sugar and albumen.
    f. *Urine culture:* During pregnancy a woman becomes more susceptible to urinary tract infections. Five percent of women have latent urinary tract infections. Because the hormone progesterone relaxes smooth muscle, the collecting area in the kidneys and the tubes connecting kidneys to bladder become larger. Urine tends to stagnate there, aggravating any latent infection. Signs of infection are frequent urination accompanied by hurting or burning. More extreme signs of infection are: back pain, chills, fever, and bloody urine.[2]

4. Regular checking of *blood pressure, weight, height of the uterus, fetal position* and *heart rate*.

5. Prescription of treatments as necessary and *vitamin and mineral* supplements.

6. During the ninth month, regular pelvic exams to check the cervix for softening, thinning, and dilatation, and to check the position of the fetus.

7. *Ultrasound:*[3] A technique using high frequency sound waves to visualize soft tissue. Ultrasound (echography, B-scan) is often used in obstetrics as well as other fields of medicine. High frequency sound waves, beyond the range of human hearing, are beamed through the pregnant woman's abdomen towards the fetus. The return

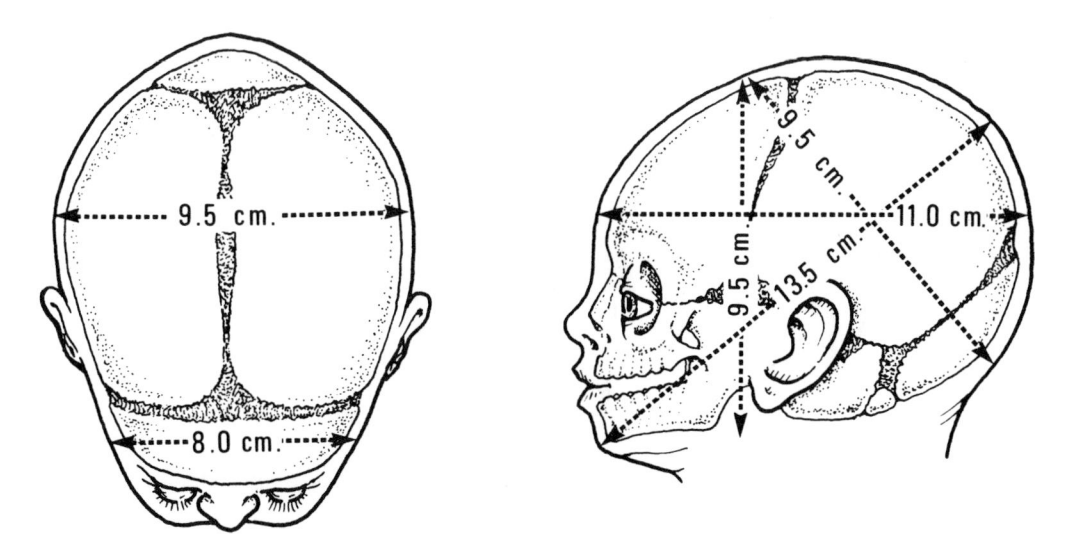

Figure 7.1. Measurements of the Fetal Head.

echo is converted to dots which can be visualized on a screen, much like a fuzzy black and white T.V. picture. Ultrasound can depict soft tissue in detail, allowing one to see the fetus and position of the placenta.

Since the sound waves are more easily conducted through liquid, the pregnant woman is instructed to drink a large amount of liquids prior to her appointment and not to urinate until after the ultrasound examination. The sound waves are beamed through the full bladder towards the uterus.

So far, ultrasound has proven very safe for mother and baby. Some doctors routinely order ultrasound while others do not. In high-risk pregnancy, frequent examinations with ultrasound may be ordered to assess fetal growth.

Information learned from ultrasound examination:

- gestational age by measurement of the fetal head (the biparietal diameter); most favourable time for this exam is 16th to 28th week of pregnancy.
- location of the placenta.
- diagnosis of twins, triplets, etc.

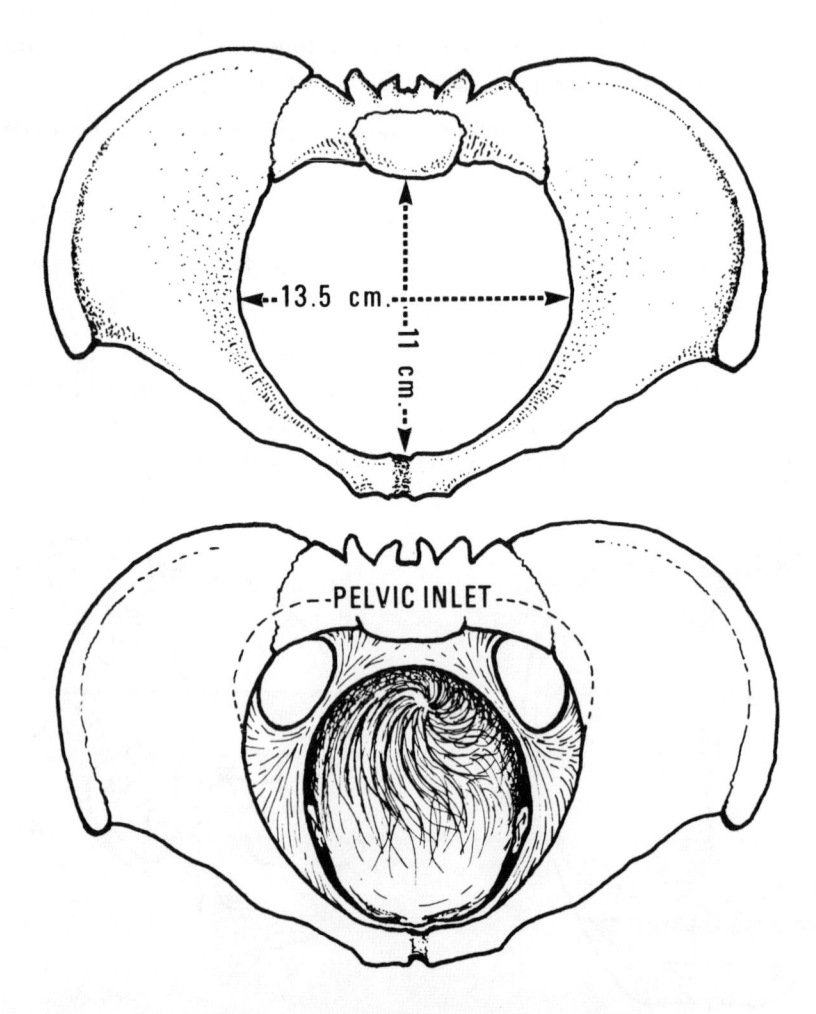

Size of baby's head vs. size of mother's pelvis.

Figure 7.2. Assessment of Cephalo-Pelvic Disproportion (CPD).

- monitoring of fetal growth, assessment for fetal growth retardation.
- detection of certain anomalies such as anencephaly, hydrocephaly, hydramnios.
- confirmation of fetal position.
- assessment of cephalo-pelvic disproportion (CPD), i.e., size of baby's head vs. size of mother's pelvis.
- used as a guide for amniocentesis.

OTHER DIAGNOSTIC PROCEDURES THAT MAY BE ORDERED

Blood Tests

Rubella Antibody Titer

If you are not immune to German measles (rubella), try to avoid exposure during pregnancy. The disease can cause miscarriage (spontaneous abortion), stillbirth, and fetal defects, although not in all cases. It's best to have a blood test prior to conception to determine whether or not you are immune to rubella. If you are not, get immunized and wait three to six months before becoming pregnant. Do not get inoculated while pregnant.

For the non-immunized pregnant woman who is exposed to rubella, gamma globulin may be given to prevent development of the disease.[4]

Coombs Test

This test is done during pregnancy on all Rh negative women. It identifies the presence of anti-Rh antibodies that can produce hemolytic (blood) disease in the Rh positive fetus.

With titers of 1 to 8 or more an amniocentesis is done at specific intervals to measure the amount of bilirubin pigment present in the amniotic fluid. Management of the Rh-negative sensitized mother is based on amniotic fluid bilirubin levels. Care may include intrauterine transfusion, induction of labour and follow-up treatment of the baby with phototherapy or transfusion.[5]

Screening for Sickle Cell Anemia

This is a hereditary blood disease that primarily affects the black population. A black person may have the disease or be a carrier of the disease. In either case, the disease can be passed on to their children. The child may then develop the disease or become a carrier, depending upon the strength of the inherited trait.

Sickle cell anemia may not be apparent at birth, as it usually surfaces between 2 and 4 years of age. It causes a variety of debilitating symptoms with periods of increased illness and remissions over the years. New treatments are being researched and many children survive to adulthood. A pregnant woman with sickle cell anemia can have serious complications during pregnancy affecting her own and the baby's health.[6]

Measurement of Blood Estriol Levels

This is done to assess fetal well-being later in the pregnancy. It is *one of the many blood tests available in assessment of mother and baby.*

Estriol is a hormone produced through interaction between the placenta and fetus and excreted in the mother's urine. Estriol levels decrease as the placental function deteriorates. Blood estriol tests can give a more accurate picture of the estriol level. Blood tests for estriols may be combined with 24-hour urine collection for measurements of estriol and creatinine.[7]

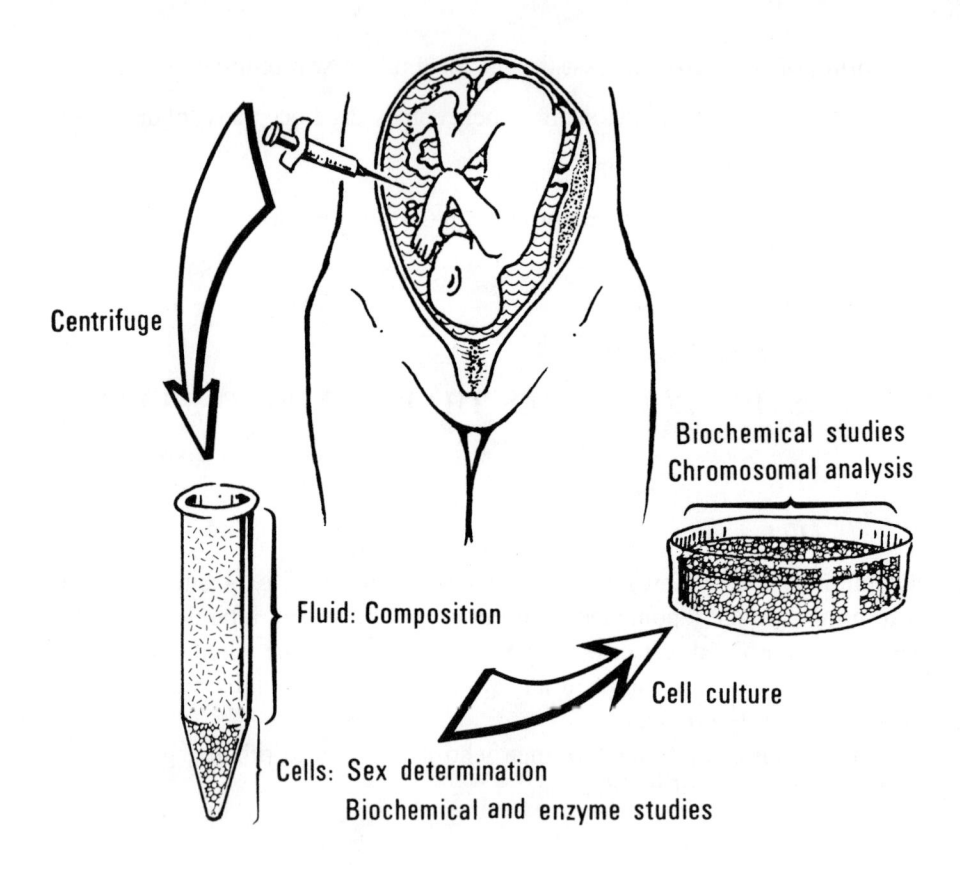

Figure 7.3. Amniocentesis.

Amniocentesis. Amniotic fluid is aspirated with a sterile syringe. Sample is centrifuged to separate cells and fluid. A variety of tests can be done.[10] Procedure performed under local anesthetic and using sterile technique.

Amniocentesis

Under local anesthetic, a needle is inserted through the abdominal and uterine walls into the amniotic cavity and a sample of fluid is withdrawn for examination. Amniocentesis is performed in early pregnancy between the 14th to 16th week when genetic problems are suspected; e.g., when there is a history of previous genetic or metabolic disorder and/or when the maternal age is 35 or older. In later pregnancy amniocentesis may be performed to assess fetal health.

Amniotic fluid derives from secretions and fetal urine and it contains fetal cells. The cells reflect the chromosomal and genetic composition of the fetus.

There are some risks to amniocentesis. In early pregnancy the amniocentesis may cause miscarriage (spontaneous abortion). Other risks include trauma to the fetus or placenta, bleeding, infection, premature labour, and Rh sensitization from fetal bleeding into the maternal circulation. The risk of amniocentesis to the mother or to the fetus is said to be in the range of 1%.[8]

Prior to amniocentesis, for whatever reason, the expectant mother should be informed of the specific risk factors and asked to sign a consent form. Information as to risk might include the following points.

1. The risk factor to mother and fetus is approximately 1%.
2. The culture of fetal cells may not be successful.
3. Repeated amniocentesis may be required.

4. Chromosome analysis, biochemical analysis, or both may not be successful.

5. Normal chromosomes results, normal biochemical results, or both, do not eliminate the possibility that the child may have birth defects or mental retardation because of other disorders.[9]

Information That Can Be Gained by Amniocentesis:

1. Observation of *Colour*: Observing the colour of the amniotic fluid will give the doctor specific information about the fetus. A bloody fluid sample cannot be used as it results in cell growth failure and changes the level of other constituents. A green sample indicates the presence of meconium (residue from the fetal intestinal tract). This is generally associated with fetal distress. At term, the amniotic fluid normally appears colourless. Earlier in the pregnancy it appears yellowish.

2. *Presence of Genetic or Metabolic Disorders*: Cells from the amniotic fluid are cultured. The chromosomes from the cells are then examined for any of the known chromosomal genetic disorders. Cultured amniotic cells are also examined for the presence of abnormal biochemical components indicating an abnormal metabolic condition in the fetus.

3. Identification of *Fetal Sex*.

4. Examination for *Alphafetoprotein*: This is a major plasma protein characteristic of early fetal life. It is produced by the fetal liver and yolk sac and can be found in amniotic fluid by radio-immunoassay. There is a marked elevation of alphafetoprotein in pregnancies associated with open neural tube defects such as spina bifida, anencephaly, etc. Amniocentesis is useful in monitoring the pregnancies of women who have had a previous baby with an open neural tube defect.

5. Measurement of *Amniotic Fluid Bilirubin*: The amniotic fluid bilirubin is measured to assess fetal health in the case of an Rh sensitized mother. Normally, during the latter half of the pregnancy, the concentration of amniotic fluid bilirubin decreases as the fetus matures. In Rh incompatibility, where the mother has developed antibodies against Rh-positive blood, bilirubin levels rise. The bilirubin level will be rechecked as the pregnancy progresses to monitor the baby's condition. The goal is to keep the baby in the uterus and to allow him to mature there as long as the environment is healthy.

6. *Lecithin-Sphingomyelin (L/S) ratio*: This is a test to assess fetal lung maturity. Mature lungs have a sticky substance called surfactant in the alveoli (air sacs). The surfactant helps prevent collapse of the lungs on expiration. Without surfactant the newborn develops respiratory distress syndrome (RDS) or hyaline membrane disease (HMD). The L/S ratio assesses two components of surfactant: lecithin and sphingomyelin. Normally, during gestation the sphingomyelin concentrations are greater than those of lecithin until about 26 weeks of gestation. From 26 to 34 weeks gestation the concentration of lecithin to sphingomyelin is approximately 1:1. From 34 to 36 weeks the lecithin rises and the ratio changes. An L/S ratio of 2:0 or greater indicates pulmonary maturity.[11]

Many other tests are performed on amniotic fluid later in the pregnancy; a few of the more common ones have been mentioned. The tests are a way of asking the baby (fetus) "How are you?" and "Would you rather be somewhere else?" (e.g., outside the uterus, born).

FETAL MONITORING[12]

Fetal monitoring is an electronic technique used to determine fetal heart rate and uterine activity. These are traced on a graph paper giving an indication of the way the fetus is tolerating labour. The baby's heart beat can also be heard, and this is reassuring to both the obstetrical staff and mother.

Fetal monitoring remains a controversial issue but is being used more and more frequently as one of the tools in assessing fetal well-being during labour. At present, in Montreal, some hospitals use continuous electronic monitoring of all women in labour; other hospitals monitor high-risk patients continuously and other patients manually at regular intervals. Often the "labour partner" (coach, husband, friend) appreciates being able to "see" the contraction and encourages the woman in labour accordingly. There are two types of fetal monitoring which may be used.

1. *External or Indirect Monitoring*: Two sensors are placed strategically on the mother's abdomen and held in place by belts. The larger sensor monitors the labour activity; the smaller, cardiac sensor, monitors the fetal heart rate. Two types of cardiac monitors are available: one type detects the actual sound of the fetal heart beat while the other type detects the movement of the fetal heart valves. To improve the contact between the mother's body and the sensor, electrode jelly is applied to the skin before the sensors are placed on the abdomen. External monitoring does limit the mother's movements as the sensors may be dislodged. If the mother is restless, internal monitoring may be chosen.

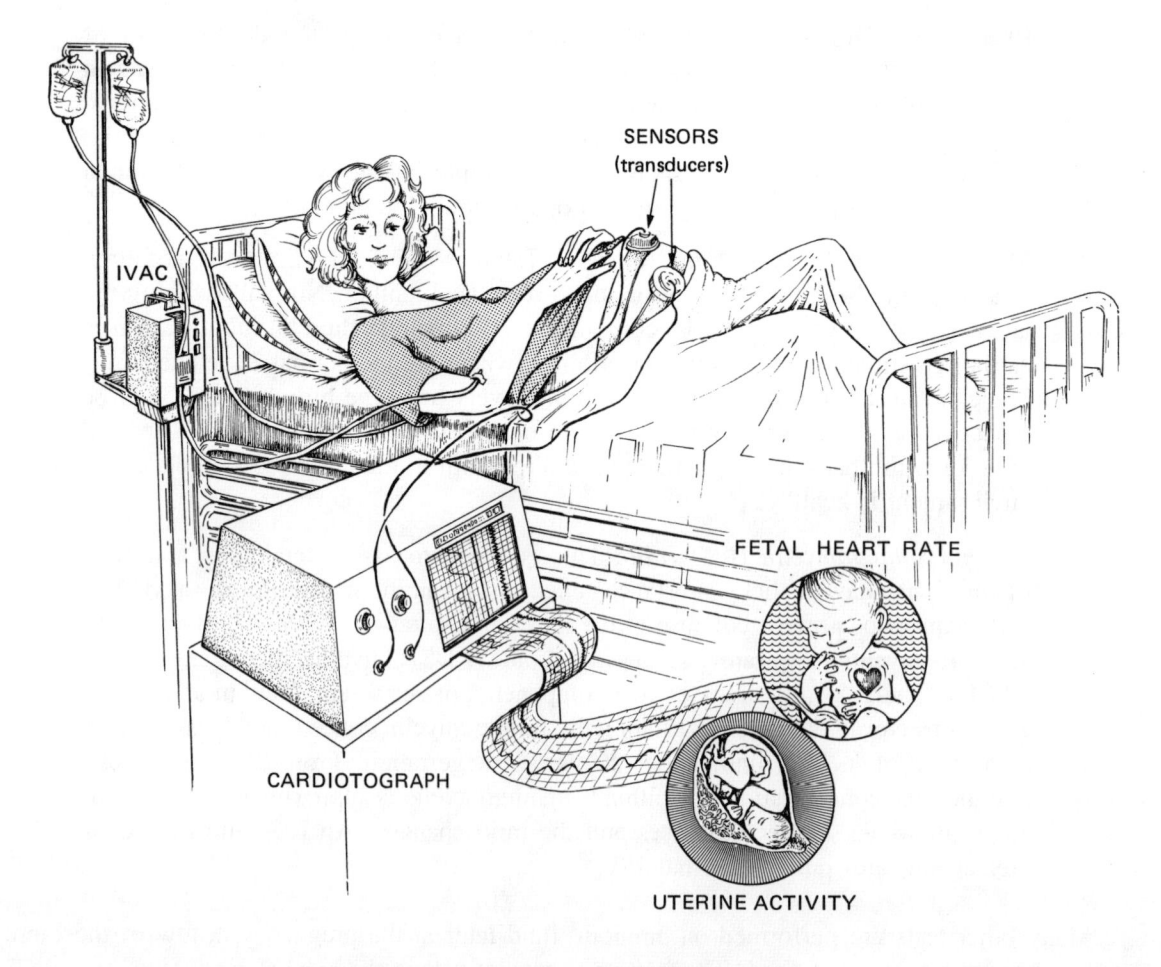

Figure 7.4. External Fetal Monitoring.

2. *Internal or Direct Monitoring*: Once the membranes have ruptured it is possible to monitor internally. This is a more accurate technique. It also allows the mother more freedom of movement. Labour activity is recorded directly by the use of a small soft plastic-tube catheter. The catheter is inserted through the vagina and into the uterus. Then it is filled with sterile water, connected to a pressure sensor, and the sensor is connected to the cardiotograph. Changes in uterine pressure are then transmitted through the fluid filled catheter to the sensor. The sensor converts the changes in pressure to electrical impulses which are measured by the cardiotograph. The fetal heart activity is recorded from a tiny electrode attached to the baby's scalp (inserted via the vagina).[13] While there are advantages to direct or internal monitoring, there is also a greater risk of infection.

NON-STRESS TEST

The non-stress test is a method used to test the normal fetal heart rate and variability; it is used to assess fetal well-being. Using the external fetal monitoring set-up. the fetal heart rate is recorded over a short period of time and fetal heart response to stimuli, such as movement of the fetus or sound, is observed. The normal fetus will produce characteristic heart rate patterns showing acceleration of the heart rate when the baby moves. The test can be done on an out-patient basis at the hospital or elsewhere. It takes approximately 30 minutes. As the name of the test implies, it is the testing of the fetal heart without any added stress, so relax. The test may be repeated several times during the last trimester; depending upon results, a Stress Test may be ordered.

STRESS TEST OR OXYTOCIN CHALLENGE TEST (OCT)

The stress test or OCT is an assessment of fetal well-being and placental function. The test monitors the fetal heart response to stress, i.e., uterine contractions. This indicates the baby's ability to tolerate labour. The OCT provides a means of assessing the degree of uteroplacental reserve. The ability of the fetus to withstand a decreased oxygen supply can be assessed by providing a physiologic stress—the uterine contraction. The healthy fetus will exhibit a reassuring fetal heart rate pattern, while the compromised fetus will demonstrate a non-reassuring pattern.

Generally the OCT is conducted by giving the pregnant woman intravenous oxytocin (pitocin, syntocinon) via an infusion pump sufficient to elicit three contractions within a 10-minute period. Simultaneously, the fetal-heart rate and uterine activity are recorded with an external monitoring set-up. The results are then interpreted.

The OCT may be started as early as 28 weeks' gestation when clinically indicated, but it is usually not done until after 34 weeks' gestation.[14]

The test is performed at the hospital on an in-patient basis. It takes an average time of two hours. Upon admission a consent form is signed; mother is asked to empty her bladder; she is assisted into a comfortable position, usually propped up in bed, and the external monitoring sensors are positioned and connected to the fetal monitor (cardiotocograph). An intravenous (IV) is started and oxytocin (syntocinon or pitocin) is given in measured amounts (via the IV) to induce the uterus to contract. A nurse remains constantly throughout the test to reassure the mother, conduct the test, and observe the effects of the test on both mother and fetus.

Use your relaxation and breathing techniques to help you relax during the test. The contractions will be mild ones and will not start your labour. (With induction for labour, a similar technique is used but with stronger doses of the medication.)

URINE ESTRIOLS

Urine estriols are used to assess placental function and fetal well-being. Estriol, as mentioned earlier, is produced by interaction between placenta and fetus. The pregnant woman may be asked to collect all her urine for a 24-hour period; a series of collections, i.e., for several 24-hour periods would be required to obtain meaningful data. The urine is then analysed for its estriol content. As the placental function deteriorates the estriol levels decrease. The test is used in conjunction with other tests.

FETAL SCALP SAMPLING

Fetal scalp sampling is used to assess the condition of the baby (fetus) during labour. This test is done in conjunction with other tests, e.g., fetal heart monitoring, maternal blood tests. Fetal distress is almost always caused by a reduced flow of oxygen-rich blood to the fetus. When the oxygen supply is depleted, the pH of the fetal blood is lowered. The pH is a measure of the acidity or alkalinity. If the level of the pH is too low in the fetal blood, it means that the baby is in danger and must be delivered immediately, perhaps by cesarean. (Low fetal blood pH can also be caused by other factors.)

Scalp sampling is done by inserting a cone-shaped speculum into the vagina, the speculum is moved against the presenting part (usually baby's head), and a tiny prick is made. A few drops of blood are taken and analysed for the concentration of oxygen, carbon dioxide, and the pH. The results aid the medical team in determining what course of action to take.[15]

CONCLUSION

The foregoing are a few of the most commonly used tests in the obstetrical medical detective work. They are presented not to frighten you, but to help you understand what is happening. Certainly not all mothers will need all of the tests mentioned. As always, the ultimate goal is to have a healthy mother and a healthy baby.

While many problems have been referred to, it *is important to remember that the majority of pregnancies* are uncomplicated (i.e., low risk) and that *the majority of babies born are healthy.*

FOOTNOTES

[1] The Boston Women's Health Book Collective, *Our Bodies, Ourselves* (Simon and Schuster, New York, Revised Edition, 1976), pp. 258–259.

[2] *Ibid.*, p. 259 footnote.

[3] Tucker, Susan M., R.N., B.S.N., *Fetal Monitoring and Fetal Assessment in High-Risk Pregnancy* (The C. Mosby Co., St. Louis, Missouri, 1978), pp. 6–30.

[4] Hotchner, Tracy, *Pregnancy and Childbirth* (Avon, New York, 1979), p. 26.

[5] Tucker, Susan, *Fetal Monitoring*, p. 37.

[6] Hotchner, Tracy, *Pregnancy and Childbirth*, pp. 28, 29.

[7] Tucker, Susan, *Fetal Monitoring*, p. 36.

[8] *Ibid.*, pp. 38, 39.

[9] *Ibid.*, pp. 38, 39.

[10] *Ibid.*, p. 49.

[11] *Ibid.*, pp. 48–58.

[12] Hewlett & Packard Medical Electronics pamphlet, *You, Your Baby and Obstetrical Monitoring* (printed in U.S.A., 1973), pp. 6–11.

[13] *Ibid.*, pp. 6–11.

[14] *Ibid.*, pp. 110–113.

[15] Hotchner, Tracy, *Pregnancy and Childbirth*, p. 244.

Chapter 8
Posture and Back Care

As pregnancy advances, the increased weight of the uterus and baby causes the centre of gravity to shift forward, and normal hormonal changes to affect the stability of joints. To compensate for this, the abdomen slumps forward, the upper torso leans back, and the weight is carried on the heels. This posture places strain on the lower back, it weakens the abdominal muscles and results in an unattractive duck-like waddle.

Lordosis (an exaggerated inward curve of the spine), and mild backache may also result if incorrect posture remains uncorrected. Thus, for comfort, good health, and a positive body image, it is essential to learn and maintain good posture.

Good Posture **Poor Posture**

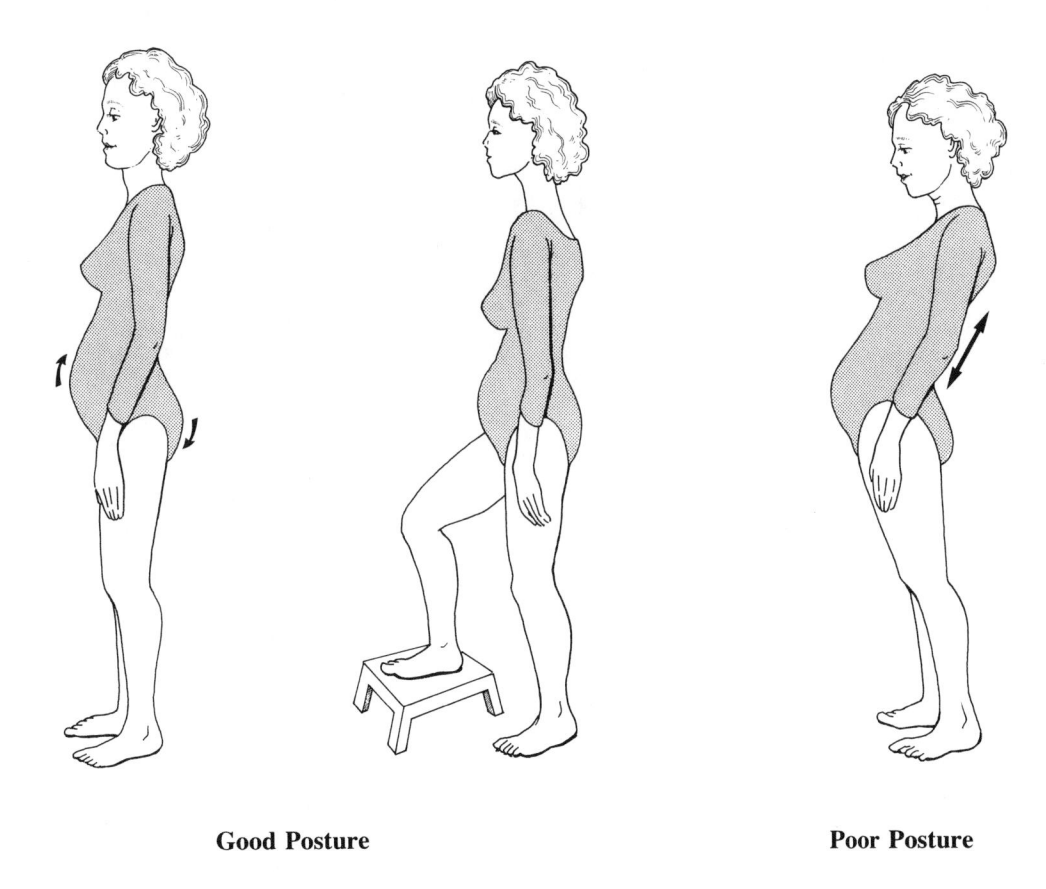

Figure 8.1. Standing.

A good standing posture may be attained by standing tall with your neck straight, and your chin tucked in, and by tilting your pelvis backward by pulling it up in the front with the abdominal muscles and down in the back with the muscles of the buttocks. In assuming this stance, you will eliminate exaggerated curvature of the spine, you will feel more comfortable and will look your best.

It is also helpful when standing for long periods of time (e.g., ironing, washing dishes) to elevate one foot by placing it on a stool or book.

Always bend from the hips and knees, never from the waist; and remember to use your legs rather than your back when lifting, if you have to lift. When lifting a heavy object, you should always bring it in close to the body, to the centre of gravity to distribute the weight evenly and avoid stressing the lower back muscles.

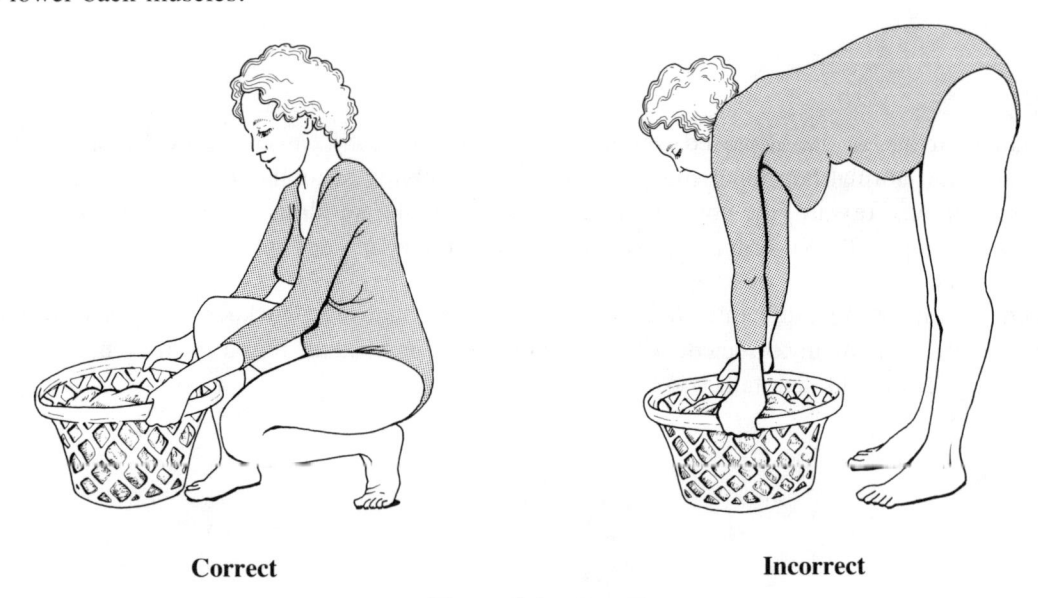

Correct   **Incorrect**

Figure 8.2. Bending.

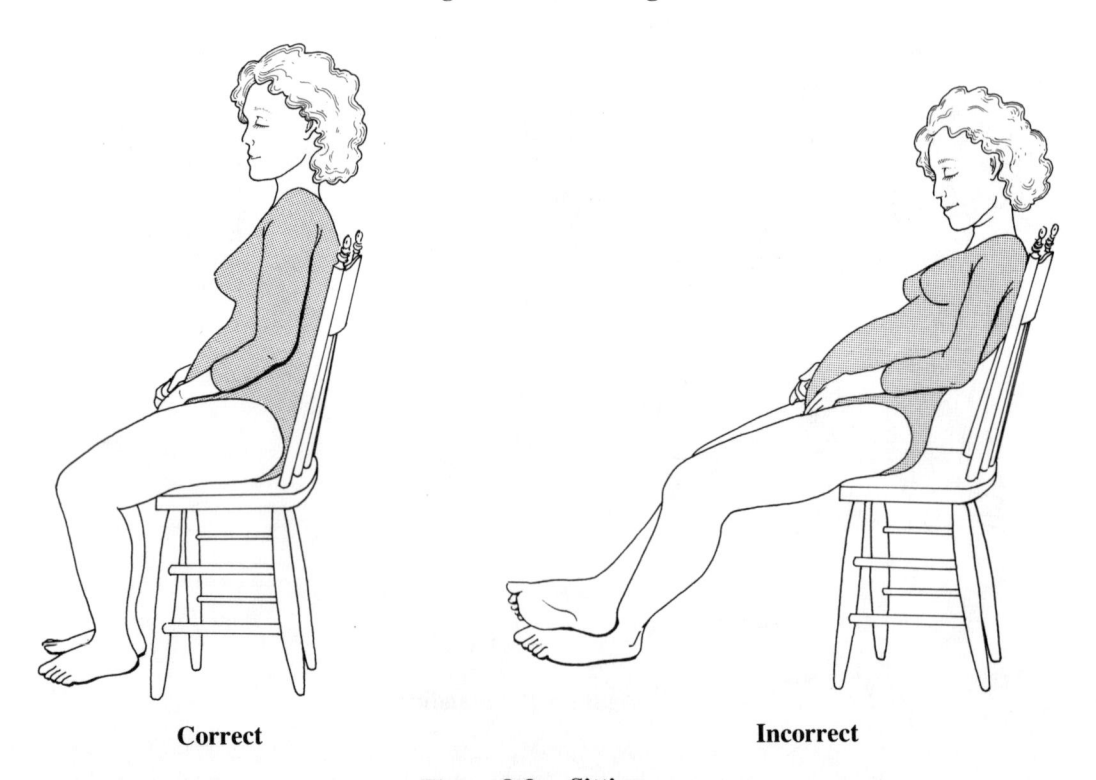

Correct   **Incorrect**

Figure 8.3. Sitting.

A good sitting position requires that your spine be well supported by the back of the chair, your knees should be even with your hips, and the entire length of your thighs should rest on the

Posture and Back Care 43

seat of the chair. For added comfort you might want to try resting your feet on a foot stool or placing pillows behind your neck or the small of your back. At all costs, avoid slouching or crossing your legs.

When lying in a supine position, it is important to eliminate the hollow in your back by placing one or two pillows under your knees. However, this position is not recommended in the later months of pregnancy because the major vessels are compressed by the weight of the baby thus lowering your blood pressure and reducing the amount of blood flowing to the placenta and baby.

A comfortable solution to this problem is the use of the side-lying position. A pillow placed lengthwise between your knees will reduce back strain and will allow you to relax.

To avoid unnecessary back strain, always use your leg muscles when rising from or lowering yourself into a chair. When rising from a lying position, turn onto your side, use your arms to lift yourself into a sitting position. From the sitting position, you progress to a squat, then push up with your legs.

Supine

Side-Lying

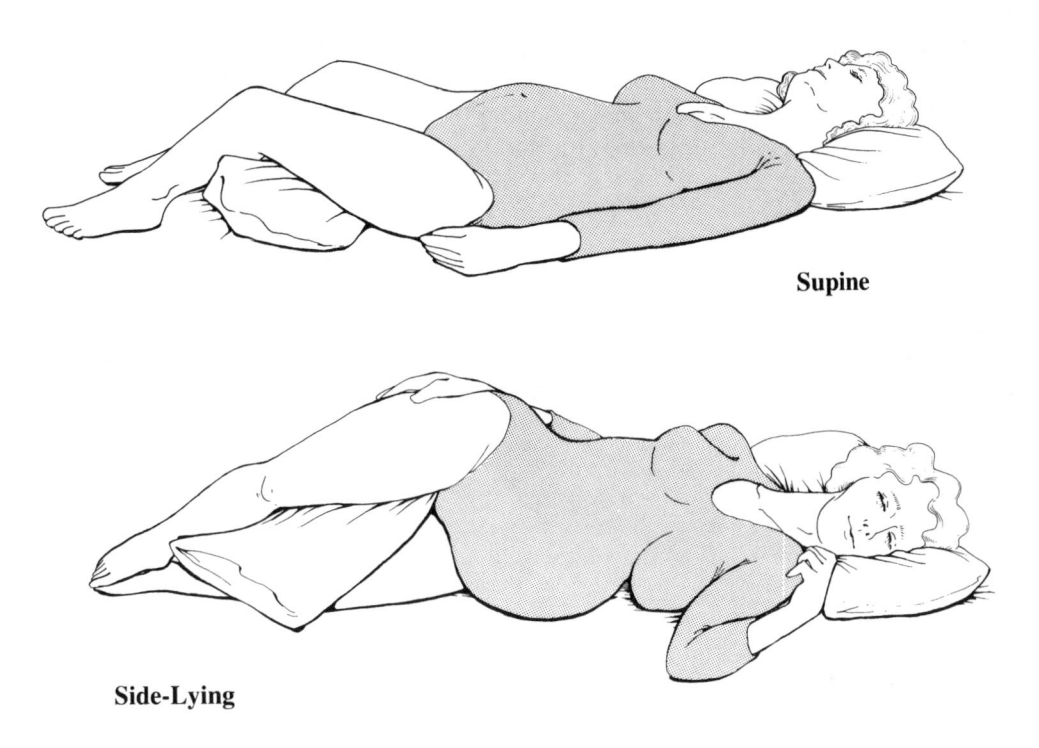

Figure 8.4. Supine and Side-Lying Positions.

Chapter 9
Prenatal Physical Exercises

During pregnancy the abdominal muscles are stretched to accommodate the increasing bulk of the uterus. At this time there is an increase in hormonal secretion which causes joints and ligaments to become lax.

It becomes important to be physically fit for the preparation for childbirth and the recovery following childbirth. Exercises are aimed at maintaining good posture as well as relieving the stresses that accompany pregnancy. Exercises will help maintain good muscular tone both prenatally and postnatally. They will help to stretch muscles in preparation for the childbearing position and will help lower extremity circulation, which may become sluggish during pregnancy.

EXERCISES

The following exercises should be performed daily. They may be continued as long as feasible. They should be done slowly and without discomfort. If discomfort or pain develops, the exercise should be discontinued. Discuss this discomfort with the doctor or childbirth educator.

1. *Trunk Reach*: This is a warm up exercise which stretches the trunk musculature.

    Method: Sit on your heels with knees slightly apart, arms resting by your sides, back straight, head bent *(position 1)*; breathe in slowly as you lift arms overhead, coming up slowly onto your knees *(position 2)*; breathe out slowly as you come back down to the resting position. Repeat 10 times.

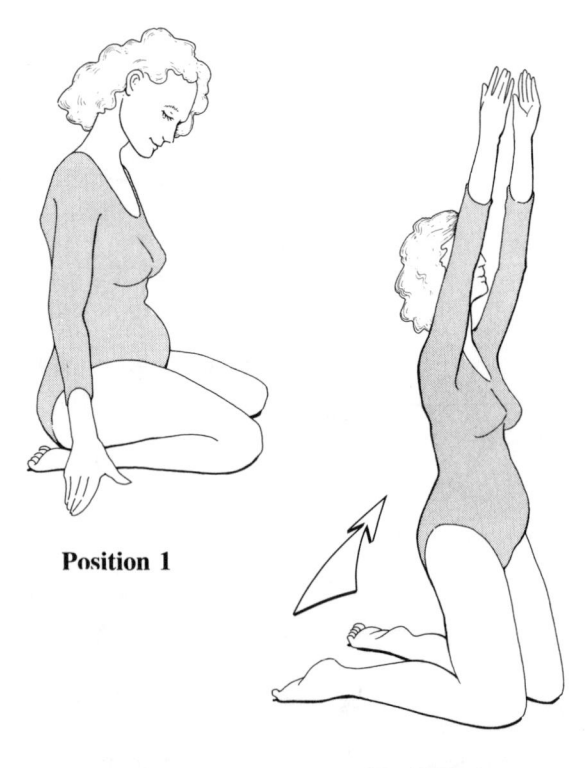

Position 1

Position 2

Figure 9.1. Trunk Reach.

Prenatal Physical Exercises 45

2. *Adductor Stretch*: This exercise will aid in stretching the inner thigh muscles and perineum in preparation for delivery.

   Method: Place soles of feet together as close to your body as possible; place hands just two inches below each knee; breathe out as you stretch knees apart and down to touch hands; breathe in as you relax. Repeat 10 times.

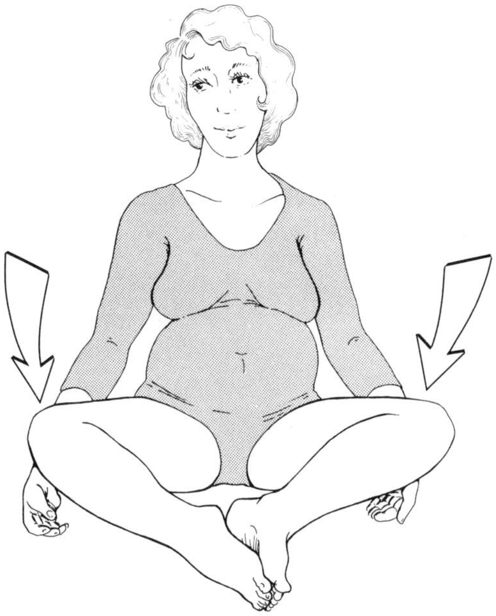

Figure 9.2. Adductor Stretch.

3. *Pectoral Exercise*: This exercise helps to strengthen the muscles supporting the breast.

   Method: Raise arms to shoulder level, palms touching; breathe out as you press hands together as hard as you can; breathe in as you relax. Repeat 10 times.

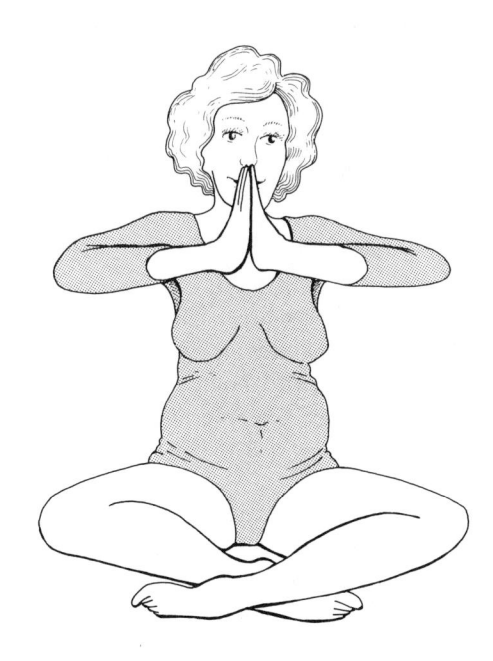

Figure 9.3. Pectoral Exercise.

4. *Pelvic Tilt*:   This postural awareness exercise will help strengthen abdominal musculature and relieve low back tension.

   Method: Lie on your back with knees bent; breathe out as you tighten your tummy, bringing your back down to touch the floor and tilting your buttocks slightly; breathe in as you relax. Repeat 10 times.

   When this exercise is mastered in the lying position, it should be practised while sitting, then standing, and finally while walking. The pelvic tilt should be your posture.

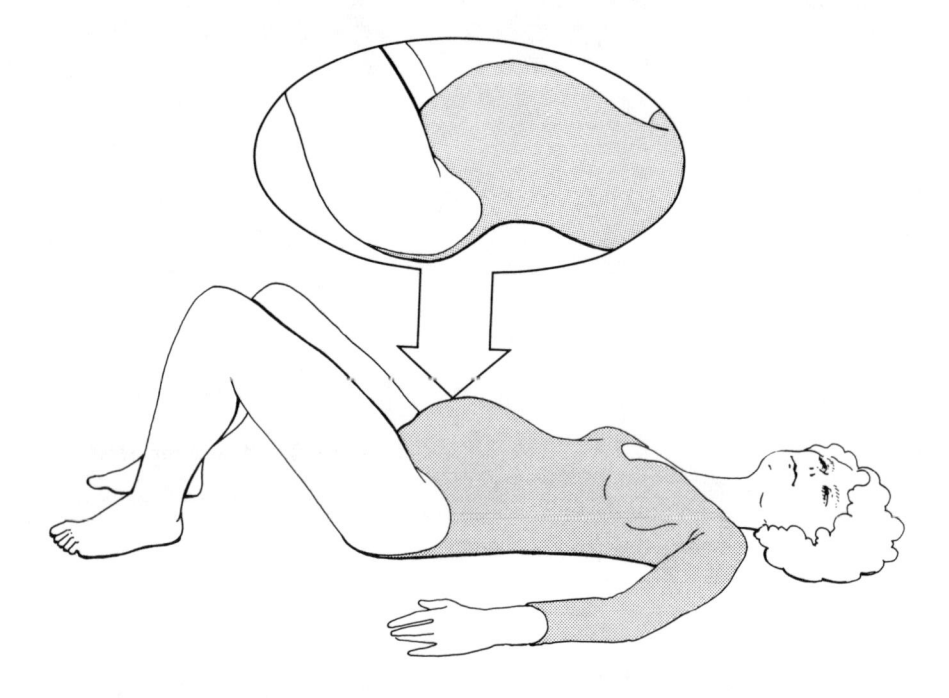

   Figure 9.4.   Pelvic Tilt.

5. *Abdominal Exercise*:   These exercises will strengthen the abdominal muscles, aid in the expulsive stage of labour, and help to restore muscular tone following childbirth.

   Method:

   Position 1:   Lie on the floor with your knees bent, tilt your pelvis as in exercise 4; breathe out slowly as you tuck your chin in, raise your head and shoulders, and stretch hands towards your knees trying to clear your shoulder blades from the floor; breathe in slowly as you lower your body to the floor. Repeat 10 times.

   Position 2:   Same as position 1, but as you raise your head and shoulders, stretch both hands to the side of your right knee; breathe in as you lower your body. Repeat 10 times.

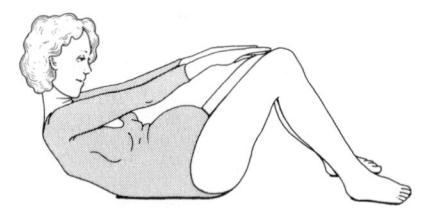

   Position 1

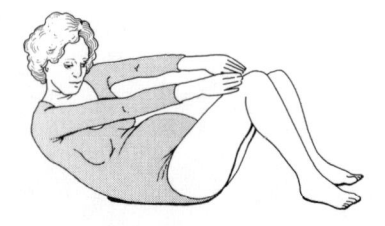

   Position 2

   Figure 9.5.   Abdominal Exercise.

Prenatal Physical Exercises 47

Position 3: Same as position 1, but as you raise your head and shoulders, stretch both hands to the side of your left knee; breathe in as you lower your body. Repeat 10 times.

Note: If, while performing the abdominal exercises you feel a soft bulge in the middle abdominal region, chances are that you are separating the rectus abdominus muscles. This may occur during the last three months of pregnancy. Although there is no danger to yourself or the baby, you should discontinue exercise 5. Concentrate instead on exercise 4 for the remaining prenatal period.

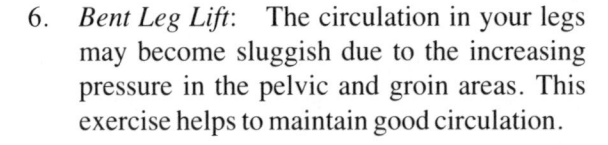

Position 3

6. *Bent Leg Lift*: The circulation in your legs may become sluggish due to the increasing pressure in the pelvic and groin areas. This exercise helps to maintain good circulation.

   Method: Lie on your back with knees bent; bend your right leg to your chest *(position 1)*; straighten the leg into the air, keeping your foot bent up (flexed) *(position 2)*; lower the straight leg slowly to the floor, then return to the bent knee position. Repeat with the left leg. Repeat 10 times.

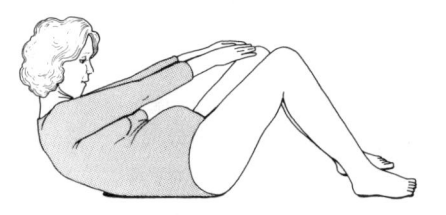

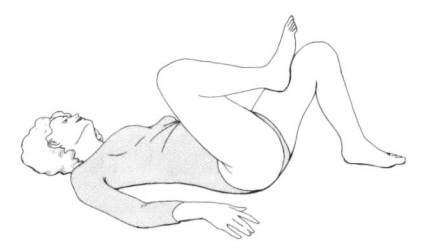

Position 1

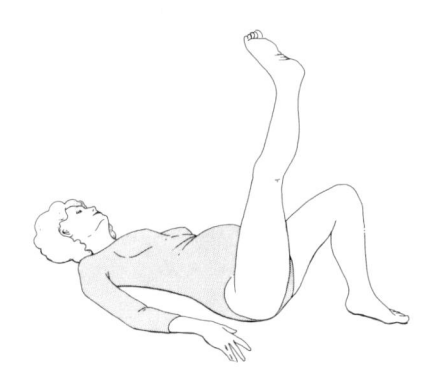

Position 2

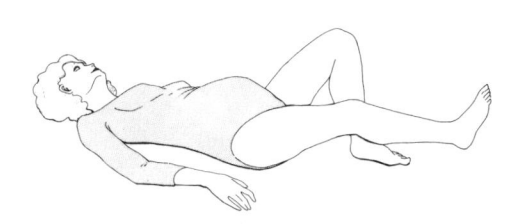

Position 3

Figure 9.6. Bent Leg Lift.

7. *Kegel Exercise*: This exercise strengthens the pelvic muscles; following childbirth it helps restore tone in the muscles supporting the bladder and uterus.

   Method: Contract pelvic floor muscles, hold 5 seconds, relax; i.e., contract or hold muscles simulating an attempt to stop urination in mid-flow. Repeat 10 times.

8. *Pelvic Tilt in 4-Point Kneel*: This exercise relieves back pressure and mobilizes the spine.

   Method: Kneel with hands on the floor, head and back straight; arch your back like a cat pulling in your tummy; breathe out as you arch; breathe in as you relax back to straight position. Repeat 10 times.

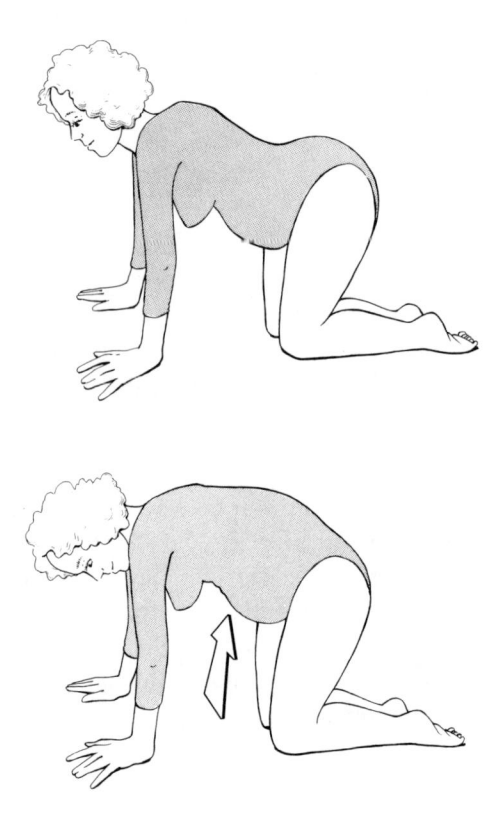

Figure 9.7. Pelvic Tilt in 4-Point Kneel.

Table 9.1. Relief of Common Aches Occurring in Pregnancy

Aches	Remedies
Loss of urine during laughter or coughing	Practise perineal exercises
Abdominal pain while coughing	Sit with feet supported and trunk inclined forward
Feeling of heaviness in the abdomen	Pelvic tilt and perineal exercises; good posture
Hemorrhoids and swelling of the vagina	Sit with feet elevated; perineal exercises; avoid constipation; avoid standing prolonged periods of time
Low back pain	Pelvic tilt exercise; practise good posture; rest (in position of relaxation); comfortable and good support shoes
Cramps in calves and toes	Movement of foot or toes in direction opposite the cramp (i.e., stretching the cramp)
Varicose veins	Elevate legs often; avoid standing prolonged periods; make circles with feet; wear support hose
Shortness of breath	Practise good posture; practise deep chest breathing; sit or semi-recline; avoid heavy meals; avoid heavy exercises
Pain in upper back	Make circles with shoulders; practise good posture; give constant pressure massage; rest frequently
Numbness in arms or fingers	Consult your doctor

For further information, consult with your childbirth educator. If any of the above symptoms persist, please consult your doctor.

SECTION II:
LABOUR AND BIRTH

Chapter 10
Relaxation

The uterus is an involuntary muscle, meaning that after a contraction starts, there is little one can do to stop the contraction. There is a tendency to tense the voluntary muscles in the whole body during a uterine contraction. You must be able to locate these tense muscle groups over which you have control, to dissociate them from the uterine contractions and to affectively reduce the tension in them.

In this way, you will remain relaxed during labour and will conserve energy. With practice, relaxation should become an automatic response to a uterine contraction; i.e., you will develop muscle control while at the same time letting the uterus do the work of contracting. The fundamental aspects of relaxation are:

1. *Comfortable position*: You cannot relax properly if you are not comfortable. The positions which favour physical relaxation are the following:
   a. Lying on your back with a pillow under the head and under the knees; the arms are resting in a relaxed position by your side.
   b. Lying on your side with a pillow under your head; the upper leg is bent and supported on pillows.
   c. Sitting in a comfortable armchair.
2. *Concentration on a Focal Point*: A focal point is any object on which you will focus during your uterine contractions, be it a spot on the wall or a favorite doll. The concentration on a focal point will prevent you from being distracted by activity about you. You will be better able to concentrate on your relaxation and breathing technique. Use the same focal point whenever you practise.
3. *Cleansing Breath*: This is a very deep breath taken in through the nose and blown out through the mouth. You will take this cleansing breath at the beginning of each contraction and at the end of each contraction. As you exhale you relax all the muscles in your body over which you have control.
4. *Knowledge of Key Areas*: These include areas such as the jaw or pelvic floor muscles. Quite often the jaw and the entire face indicate muscle tension elsewhere in the body. By concentrating on key areas, you enhance relaxation in the arms and legs. After taking the cleansing breath concentrate on relaxing the key areas.
5. *Participation of Coach*: Verbal cues or reinforcements during a contraction such as "contraction begins" or "cleansing breath" enhances your concentration. Also, the coach provides comfort measures such as effleurage to help you remain relaxed.

CONDITIONS FAVOURING RELAXATION

The practice of special relaxation techniques should be done at first in a well-ventilated and calm area. When you feel at ease with the techniques, practise relaxing in different situations such as at work, at the dentist, in the car, during a traffic jam, etc. Remember that the hospital will not be a quiet and calm place.

The ultimate goal is to achieve neuromuscular control in labour, that is, to gain a willed control (through practice) of all voluntary muscles which may develop useless tension during labour.

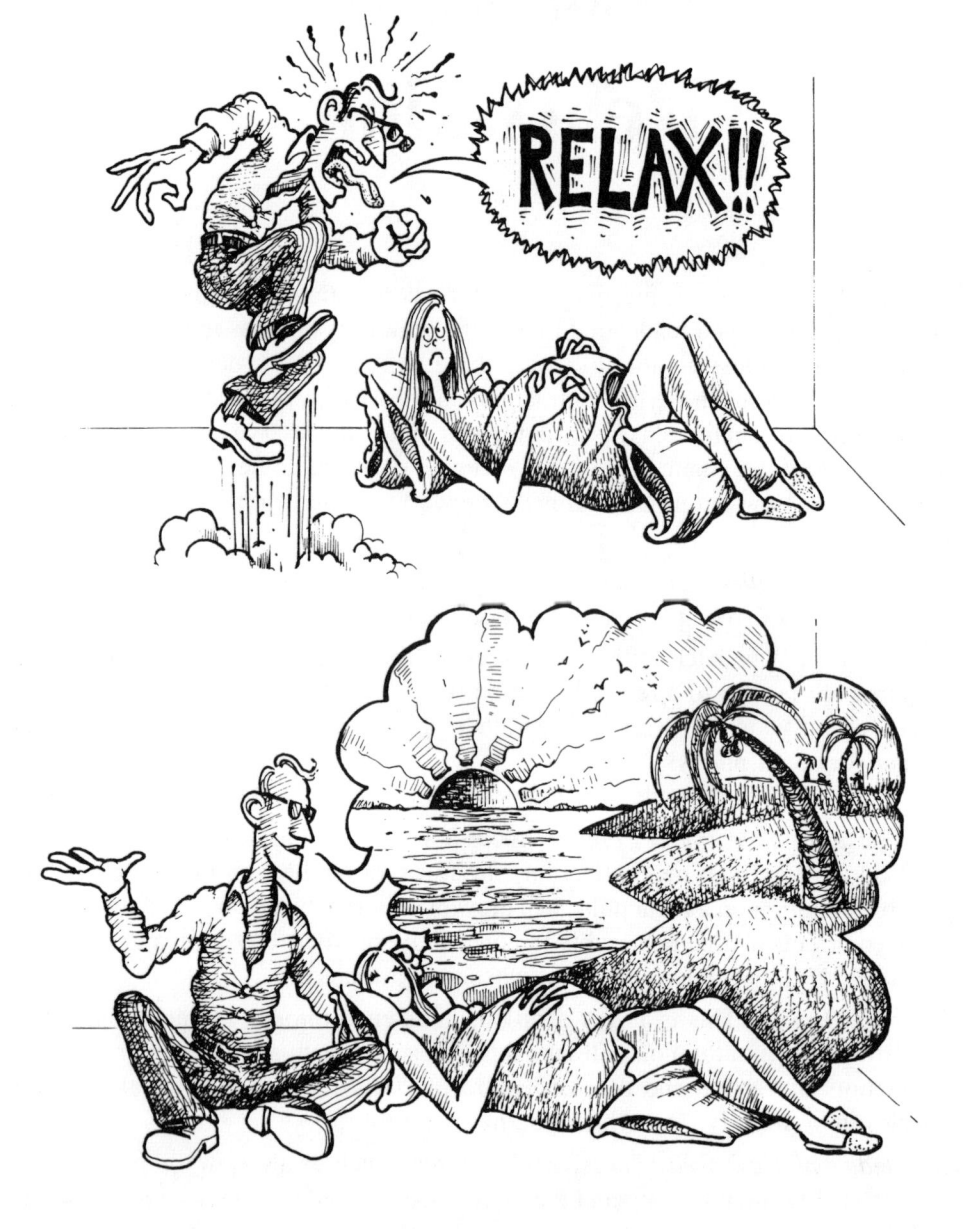

Participation of Coach.

TECHNIQUES OF RELAXATION

1. Repeat three contractions of each muscle group (legs, arms, trunk and head, and face) as follows, from a maximal contraction to a minimal. For example, in tightening your arm you will:
    a. Tighten or contract your arm maximally. Relax.
    b. Tighten or contract your arm less strongly. Relax.
    c. Tighten or contract your arm slightly. Relax.
2. Relax gradually after each contraction. Be attentive and concentrate on the state of relaxation produced after each contraction.
3. Precede and end each contraction with a deep cleansing breath.

Relaxation 55

The Legs

1. Pull your right foot towards your head.

   Example of Techniques

   a. Take a deep cleansing breath.
   b. Pull your right foot towards your head as hard as you can. Hold for three seconds.
   c. Relax gradually.
   d. Take a deep cleansing breath.
   e. Pull your right foot towards your head with moderate force. Hold for three seconds.
   f. Relax gradually and take another cleansing breath.
   g. Pull your right foot towards your head with minimal force. Hold for three seconds.
   h. Relax and take another deep cleansing breath.

   Repeat with the opposite foot.

2. Pull your right foot towards your head, and push the knee towards the floor. Repeat with the left leg.

3. Pull your right foot towards your head, knee down, tighten thigh and hip muscles (i.e., keep the tension in the entire leg). Repeat with the left leg.

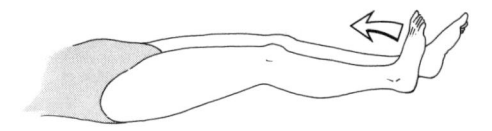

Position 1

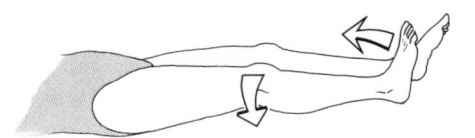

Position 2

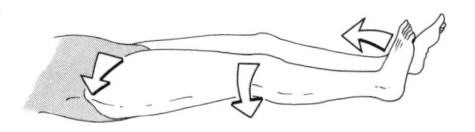

Position 3

Figure 10.1. The Legs.

The Arms

1. Make a fist with the right hand. Repeat with the left hand.

2. Make a fist and straighten the elbow, and press the right arm down into the floor (i.e., keep the tension in the entire arm). Repeat with the left arm.

Position 1

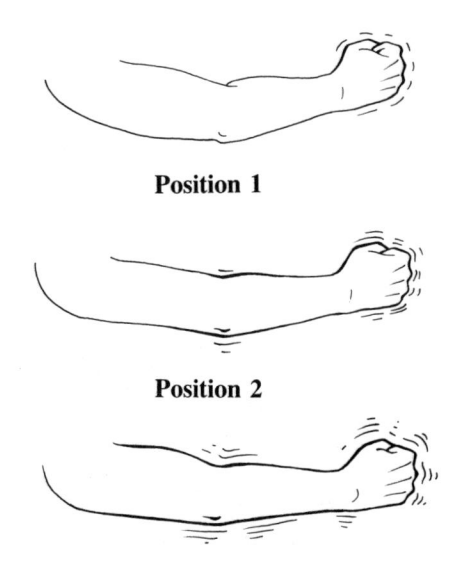

Position 2

Position 3

Figure 10.2. The Arms.

The Trunk and Head

1. Squeeze together your buttocks and tighten your abdominals.

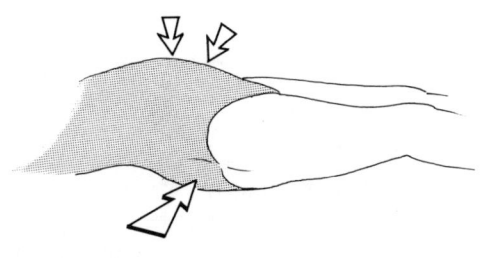

2. Lift your shoulders towards your ears.

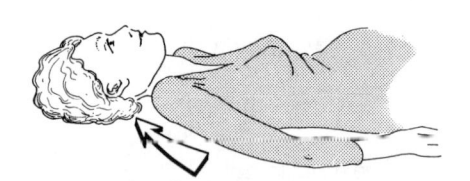

3. Press your shoulders towards the floor squeezing shoulder blades together.

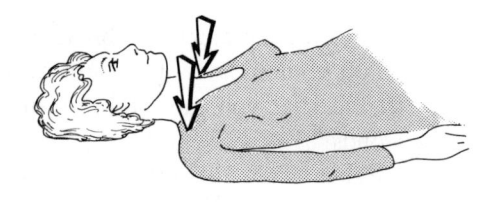

4. Keeping your chin tucked in, press your head towards the floor.

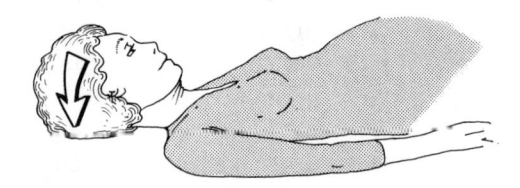

Figure 10.3. The Trunk and Head.

The Face

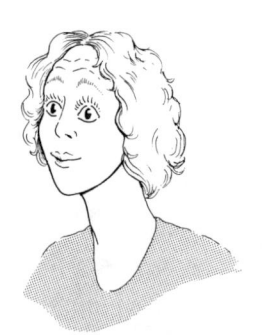

1. Lift your eyebrows, wrinkling your forehead.

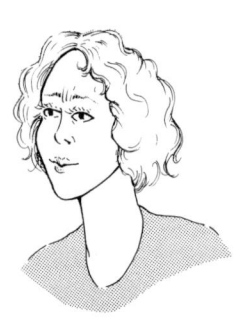

2. Squeeze your eyebrows together.

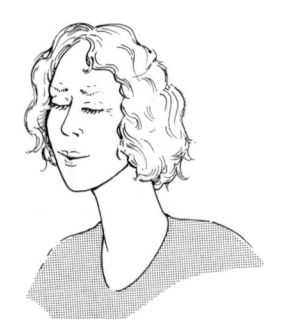

3. Squeeze your eyes closed.

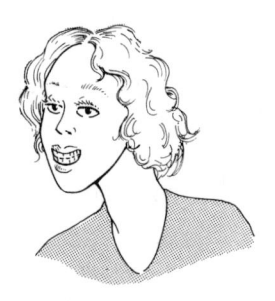

4. Clench your teeth.

Figure 10.4. The Face.

By practising the above drills you will recognize the tension which may develop in different areas of the body. During actual labour, where the uterus is "in tension," you will not allow yourself to become tense, concentrating instead on relaxing all the muscles over which you have control.

To practise this dissociation of tension in the body, you will tense one part of the body while learning to concentrate on relaxing the rest. For example, tense your right leg as you have already practised. As you hold this tension in your leg you should be completely relaxed in the rest of your body. The coach may check for this relaxation by gently rolling the other leg or arm. Practise these dissociation drills in progressively more complicated patterns; i.e., tense right leg, tense right leg and right arm, tense left leg and right arm.

Practise until you feel at ease with these drills. Only then can you relax in labour while letting the uterus do the work. Do not attempt to practise all the above drills in one session, but take one area of the body at a time. Remember also the few fundamental points of relaxation as already mentioned.

Chapter 11
Labour

The labour process leading to the birth of a child remains one of the most rewarding, exciting, and memorable of all events. To a woman, the birth of her first child is a spectacular moment, every change in labour is important in order to bring her baby into the world.

Normal labour has a spontaneous onset and progresses by the natural, unaided efforts of the mother. The fetus (presenting by the head), and placenta, and the membranes are expelled via the birth canal at approximately forty (40) weeks. The usual length of time is 12 to 14 hours for a woman having her first child and 8 to 10 hours for a woman having her second or later children.

The onset of labour is the result of hormonal, nervous system, circulatory, and physiological changes. Labour is influenced by the powerful contractions of the muscle of the uterus (womb). The

Table 11.1. Differentiating True and False Labour

	True Labour	False Labour
Contractions	at regular intervals	are irregular
	gradual shortening of the intervals	intervals do not shorten
	increasing intensity	no change in intensity
	are intensified by walking	walking has no effect or may relieve contractions
	seem to originate in the back	origin mainly in abdomen
	quite often felt as strong menstrual cramps	
Cervix	effacement and dilatation begin as labour progresses	no effacement or dilatation
Show	usually present	never present
	small to moderate amount of blood-tinged mucus from vagina	
Membranes	may or may not be ruptured; i.e., often remain intact until labour is well-advanced	unlikely to be ruptured
	be sure to note time membranes rupture, quantity and colour of fluid draining	

pelvis is a bony ring made up of your two hip bones, sacrum, and tailbone. The pelvis must be large enough for the head of the fetus to pass through in order to provide a safe delivery. The fetus presents by the head in 96 percent of all labours. The size, position, and presentation of the fetus in relation to the mother's pelvis determines the progress made and the outcome of the labour. *Engagement* occurs when the widest diameter of the head has descended midway into the pelvis.

THE STAGES OF LABOUR

The first stage of labour is divided into three phases: the *early latent phase*, the *active phase*, and *transition*. The *early latent phase of labour* occurs from the onset of regular uterine contractions until effective dilatation of the cervix occurs (0 to 4 centimeters). The *active phase* of labour occurs from 4 cms dilatation and continues to 8 cms dilatation. *Transition* lasts from 8 cms dilatation to 10 cms or full dilatation of the cervix.

The *second stage of labour* lasts from full dilatation of the cervix until the baby is born.

The *third stage of labour* lasts from the birth of the baby until the placenta is completely delivered.

During the normal third stage of labour the cervix is soft and relaxed, and allows easy passage of the placenta as it separates from the wall of the uterus into the vagina.

Table 11.2. Duration of Labour

Phase	1st Baby	2nd Baby
Average latent phase	8.6 hours	5 hours
Maximum latent phase	20 hours	14 hours
Active phase (including transition)	5.8 hours	2.5 hours
Cervical dilatation	1.2 cms/hr.	1.5 cms/hr
Average second stage	1 hour	20 minutes

Women often ask, "How shall I prepare for labour? What should I expect?" Others say, "Describe the birth or talk about the baby." In reality they are seeking more information or reinforcement of basic but important facts related to labour and delivery.

EXTERNAL SIGNS TO LOOK FOR WHEN LABOUR STARTS

Show: this is the passage of the mucus plug from the cervix, with loss of blood-stained fluid. During pregnancy, the mucus plug was a protective barrier to infection from the vaginal route; as the cervix dilates, the mucus plug gradually comes away, not only at the outset of labour but also during active labour. You should note the time of the "show" as this may be seen many times before the birth.

Ruptured Membranes: the amniotic sac or "bag of waters" contains amniotic fluid which surrounds the fetus in the uterus. The fluid maintains equal pressure around the fetus and is protective in its function. At some point before or during labour the sac may rupture and allow amniotic fluid to leak out. The loss of amniotic fluid usually causes stronger contractions because there is direct contact of the muscle of the uterus on the baby.

The normal colour of amniotic fluid is clear. Always inform your doctor immediately when this occurs, remembering the time and colour of the fluid. It is important that you set out to the hospital at once so that you may be examined. A pelvic exam will verify the position and presentation of the fetus and the dilatation of the cervix. The fetal heart sounds should be listened to frequently.

Contractions: the onset of regular, rhythmic contractions usually convince most women that they are in labour. However, contractions become progressively stronger, are of longer duration and greater intensity. There are several terms which will help you in understanding and discussing your contractions.

The *duration* of a contraction is the interval of time from the beginning to the end of the contraction.

The *intensity* is the strength of the contraction. A contraction is usualy stronger at the end than at the outset. An ascending curve is noted in the first half of its duration and a descending curve in the second half.

The *frequency* of your contractions is the time it takes each contraction to occur; e.g., every three minutes.

The *resting phase* is the time between contractions when the uterus is at rest. At this time there should be complete relaxation of your body.

There are certain signs associated with contractions that a woman may be aware of:

- hardening of the uterus
- change in shape of the uterus
- fetal movement
- backache
- increase in fetal heart rate

Most women observe at the beginning of labour that contractions are usually mild and irregular: one in 30 minutes; one in 15 minutes, even as close as every 10 minutes.

- *Mild* contractions last approximately 20 to 35 seconds and are less frequent than 5 to 10 minutes.
- *Moderate* contractions last 40 to 50 seconds and often return within 5 minutes or less.
- *Strong* contractions may last 60 to 90 seconds or more. Such contractions usually are as frequent as 1 to 2 or 1 to 3 minutes and are very effective.

The average woman is usually in the company of her attendants in the hospital or a birthing room when her contractions are moderate to strong. Some women start labour observing just one or two of the three important signs; occasionally, a woman may have noted all three in the first few hours of labour (that is, show, ruptured membranes, and contractions).

PREPARATION FOR THE HOSPITAL

Your suitcases for mother's belongings and for baby should be packed and ready at least two weeks prior to your due date. Sometimes you may be surprised to find that you have started your labour one or two weeks early. Others may be just on time, or one or two weeks late. In hospital units where a great deal of space and accommodation affords a private room for each patient, you may bring your own suitcase with you. Where such accommodation is not possible, both suitcases may be left at home and only brought to the postpartum ward following the birth of the baby. You may bring a small bag containing:

- toothbrush and paste
- brush and comb
- cream or lotion
- talcum powder
- chap stick or lip gloss
- 2 face cloths
- lollipop or hard candy
- book to read
- games to play
- 1 or 2 extra pillows
- camera (no flash)
- money for phone calls
- sanitary belt
- sanitary pads
- slippers and housecoat

CARE OF THE MOTHER IN LABOUR

You should be fasting from the time you know that you are in labour. If you are hungry, ice chips, sips of water, and some clear fluids may be allowed, but *no* solids.

In the hospital, a one-to-one nurse/patient relationship is provided. This is necessary for effective support in normal labour. Your attendant should always identify himself or herself. All procedures should be explained and your consent obtained prior to being carried out by doctor or nurse. Care should be taken to ensure your privacy and safety.

ON ARRIVAL AT HOSPITAL

Always enter the hospital or maternity unit by the front door. At most hospitals *all* patients need to stop at the admitting office. There, certain forms will be completed as per hospital policy.

A porter escorts you to the labour room in a wheelchair. Your husband may be asked to remain in the waiting room for approximately 5 to 10 minutes while the nurse admits you.

ASSESSMENT

The nurse helps you to undress, weighs you, and obtains a specimen of urine for routine analysis (especially albumen and sugar). When you have been put to bed, the nurse does a full abdominal examination, inspection, palpation, and listens to the fetal heart. A general assessment is also made; your temperature and blood pressure are recorded. The pulse and respiratory rates are also recorded.

A brief history of the onset of labour is taken and a physical examination is performed by the doctor. Your records will be reviewed for the following: blood tests; results of X-rays and ultrasound tests; post-medical and obstetrical history; and operations performed.

Following your general assessment, the nurse and doctor continue to observe your progress in labour and meet your needs as they arise. A team spirit is favoured, encouraging an ongoing rapport between doctor, nurse, husband, and patient from the time of admission. This fosters relaxation in the mother and increases her confidence in those caring for her.

During the initial waiting period, your partner will be asked to change into his labour and delivery suit before entering the labour ward. Partners should always let the staff know that they have attended childbirth education classes and would like to assist as much as possible. Partners may stay during the physical examination or pelvic examination if they so desire. When your doctor has consulted about your admission, a "mini" shave of the pubic hair or perineal area (2 cm. in diameter) may be done and, if necessary, an enema will be given by the nurse in preparation for normal labour.

FIRST STAGE

The first stage of labour is understood as the onset of regular, rhythmic contractions (approximately every 10 minutes or less) with resultant or accompanying dilatation of the cervix from 0 to 10 centimeters.

The couple must communicate in every sense of the word, with both partners sharing the breathing and relaxation exercises. Learn to relax completely between contractions; partners should check their wives only when necessary. Social skills and background influence a couple's behaviour and self-control.

Touching is a normal expression and is often more effective than words. Massage is soothing and a basic stimulus for relaxation. Specific massage of the abdomen (effleurage), back, and thighs is appreciated by the mother. A partner should do only those things that his wife enjoys, since the aim is to achieve comfort.

Position

In early labour (0 to 4 centimeters), if membranes are intact, a woman can walk around, play games, read, and engage in other pleasant activities.

Most women feel more comfortable in the upright position, whether standing or sitting. The fetal heart rate is more stable and more progress is made due to better contractions. Positions in bed may include squatting or sitting upright, using sandbags and pillows for support. If lying flat, mother should be in the lateral position. Changing one's position often is important to avoid depressing the circulation in certain parts of the body. While in bed, leg exercises can still be done; e.g., making the letters of the alphabet with each foot. The woman should never lie on her back unless the doctor or nurse instructs her to do so.

Active

As the woman approaches the active phase of labour, the individual attention of her partner and nurse is more meaningful. She wants company and support. All couples should know:

- what is available
- what is possible
- how to ask for it
- how to respond to others and express their needs

In active labour the woman needs to concentrate more. When contractions start, she will do some breathing: i.e., shallow chest breathing or rhythmic chest breathing. As labour advances she perspires more and the back of the throat becomes dry. The husband's encouragement and praise is always welcomed. He may offer ice chips for her to suck on; he may apply counter-pressure to the lower back, especially in back labour. Lip gloss applied to the lips prevents chapping. True expressions of one's feelings and eye contact are best for the couple and allows attendants to meet their needs satisfactorily. The fetal heart sounds may be listened to continuously or intermittently, depending on the type of monitor used or the requirements of each individual labour.

Transition

Transition is the period from 8 to 10 centimeters dilatation of the cervix. Most women have mixed feelings (not an accurate sense of direction) due to the emotional turmoil of transition. Unswerving support from partner and hospital staff is needed. Light breathing is best. Mother should be encouraged to blow out instead of pushing prematurely. Shallow, quick breathing is also effective at this stage for some women. For some women, it is difficult to maintain control during the transition phase; much reinforcement is necessary for a woman to "hold on" to the end.

SECOND STAGE

At this stage, the cervix is completely dilated; that is, 10 centimeters. In speaking to many women, a variety of sensations have been reported. For example: I feel pressure in the back (rectal); stretching of tissue; tingling heat on the perineum; I feel I am opening up below (cervix fully dilated); I am sitting on something (baby's head); and I have to "push" or bear down.

Childbirth is an intense clinical and psycho-sexual experience. At this point in normal labour, a woman feels that she must respond to each wave of the contraction. The guidance of a strong partner or nurse at this time is important. Eye contact and simple sentences, and directions requiring "yes" and "no" answers are preferred. A squatting position is automatically adopted by many women.

Most women feel a sense of relief when they actually start pushing with contractions. Sometimes at full dilatation there is a resting phase of ten minutes or more when a woman does not feel like pushing immediately. Attending staff should wait for the uterine message to push. The patient may use "deep breathing" through a relaxed, open mouth and jaw. The woman's body should be completely relaxed when there are no contractions. Prolonged breath-holding decreases the blood flow to the baby and can lead to fetal distress. Therefore, it should be discouraged.

To see the baby's head advancing via an overhead mirror is both fascinating and encouraging to the couple, since the end is in sight. The husband's face may be used as a focal point in the delivery room. The woman should listen for verbal cues regarding expulsive pushing techniques. The nurse or doctor feels contractions and gives directions to push, if the mother has an epidural anesthesia and does not feel her own contractions.

Other than the patient and her husband, the people in the delivery room will include the obstetrician and his assistant and your nurse. The pediatrician may also be present if there is any concern about the baby.

The nurse positions the patient with a firm board under the mattress of the delivery bed to support her head, neck, and back. She then places the woman's feet in stirrups, if required, and cleanses the pubic and perineal area in preparation for the birth.

The doctor and assistant wear a hat, mask, sterile gown, and gloves. The husband and nurse wear a hat, mask, and labour outfit. Overshoes are also worn by all persons in the delivery room. Some hospitals are moving away from strict sterile techniques and they deliver the baby in a much more relaxed atmosphere, with street clothes for the husband and no mask and hat. The doctor places sterile drapes on the patient's abdomen, thighs, and under her buttocks. He then checks the position of the baby by pelvic examination. When there is a contraction, the patient:

1. Keeps her seat flat on the bed;
2. Pulls up on the supports or handles on either side;

3. Takes one or two cleansing breaths;

4. Breathes in "and pushes" through partially opened mouth.

5. She pushes down and out, following the curve of the birth canal. For each contraction perhaps only two or three pushes may be possible, depending on the duration of the contraction.

As the baby's head is more visible the doctor controls the birth of the head, protecting the perineum. The back of the head crowns, then the face and the head is delivered slowly. The doctor now slowly delivers the anterior shoulder, then the posterior shoulder, and gradually the whole body slips out and a child is born!

The newborn may be allowed to lie on the mother's abdomen to facilitate "bonding" and contact. The father should wash his hands and be prepared for this special moment also. The baby may be laid on the doctor's lap or held upside down to aid drainage of mucus from the nose and mouth. Mother and father should always ask to see and touch their baby and enjoy their first greeting.

Many babies have a "blue" tinge at the extremities, but with stimulation this is soon replaced by a lovely pink colour in a few minutes. In some hospitals the baby is kept in a warm crib, others in incubators. Newborn babies are very sensitive and have to be well-wrapped at all times. The preference for incubators is related to external temperature in different countries (in cold countries the babies would be kept in incubators initially).

Commonly, cord pulsation is allowed for 60 seconds—then the cord is clamped and divided. This marks the end of the second stage of labour. At this point, the woman is ecstatic and can only think of her baby, questions usually coming one after another. "What sex is the baby? Are all the organs present? What colour are the baby's eyes? What is his weight, length?" and so on.

Some time should be given for the nurse to relate all these findings. Identification bands are placed on the baby, one on each wrist, after checking with the parents for correct spelling of their name. The sex, date, name of patient, doctor, and number are printed on the wristlet.

An assessment of the health of the baby is made by the obstetrician, nurse, or pediatrician, if present. The assessment is called the apgar score and is based on the infant's colour, heart rate, respiration, muscle tone, and reflexes. Two points are awarded for each satisfactory observation, with 10 being the highest total. The apgar score of the newborn is normally between 7 and 10 in 1 to 5 minutes. Other general observations are carried out to exclude abnormalities; the doctor will also check to see how the baby is crying.

THIRD STAGE

The third stage lasts from the birth of the baby until the placenta or afterbirth has separated from the uterine wall and is completely expelled via the vagina.

Some doctors instruct the nurse to give syntocinon, 5 to 10 units, with birth of the anterior shoulder or after the placenta is expelled to encourage the uterus to contract and to reduce unnecessary blood loss. Others give no medication at all, but wait approximately five to ten minutes to allow the placenta to be delivered unaided.

The placenta is about one-sixth of the baby's weight, one to one and one-quarter pounds. The placenta is examined for its completeness and health of tissue by the obstetrician. A gentle pelvic examination is done by the doctor to ensure that there are no cervical or vaginal lacerations. Externally, the vulva and perineum are examined for bruising and lacerations. If an episiotomy was made or a small tear sustained, it would be repaired with self-absorbent sutures. When the perineum is intact, no suturing is required. Vulval cleansing is done and sterile pads are placed in position. Mother is

Complete extension (crowning)

Restitution (external rotation)

Delivery of anterior (top) shoulder

Delivery of posterior (bottom) shoulder

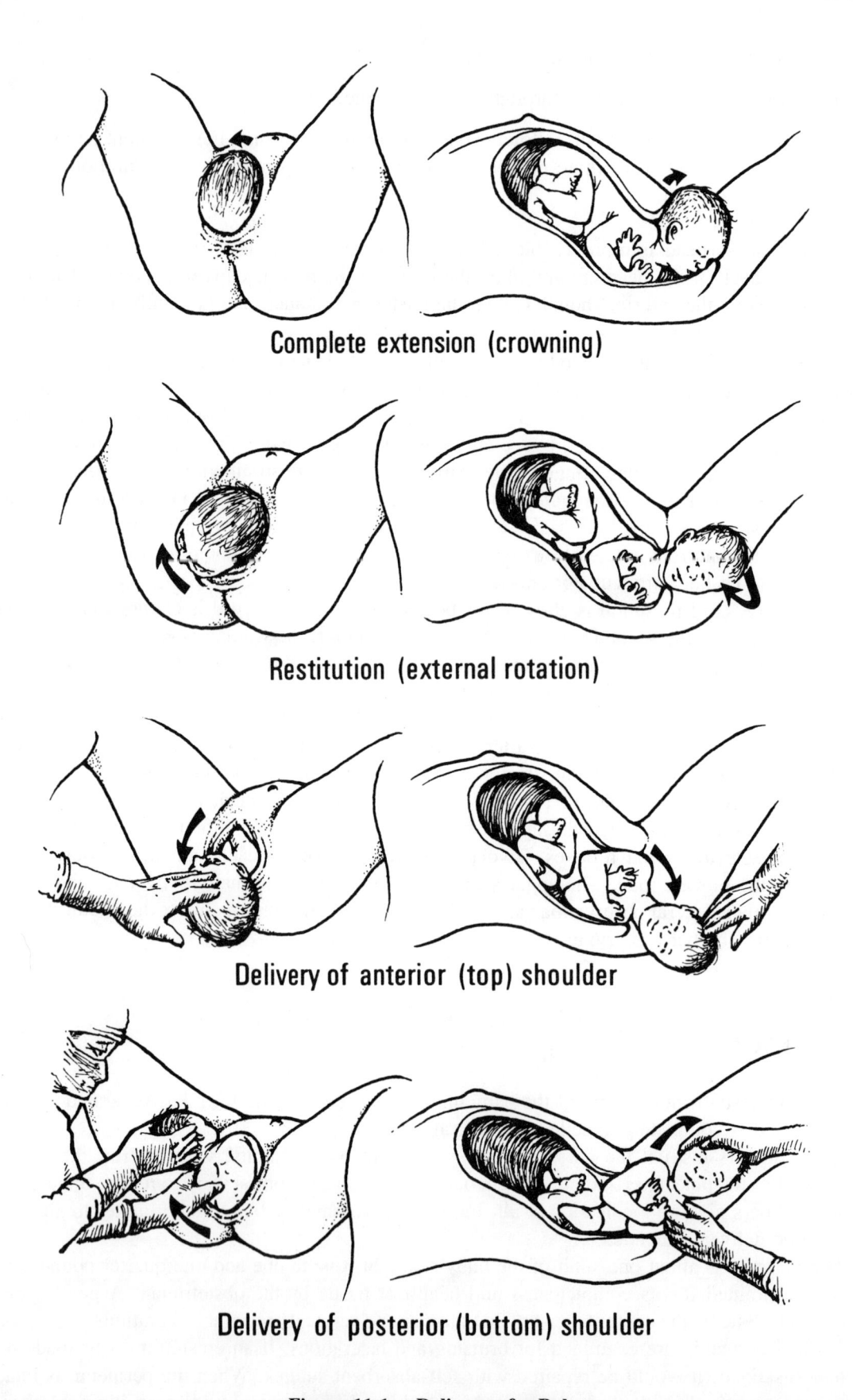

Figure 11.1. Delivery of a Baby.

made comfortable and returned to a clean bed; the baby is wrapped in warm, clean blankets and placed in her arms.

Mother and father are allowed to enjoy their baby for a while before the nurse takes the baby to the nursery to be weighed, bathed, and checked. Mother is then allowed to relax in the recovery room for one hour. Happy fathers are now free to make phone calls and have a meal while mother is being bathed and refreshed.

Three reactions are usually evident in women following the birth. The mother is very tired and just wants to sleep; or she is extremely hungry; or she is super excited, almost "walking on air," and really does not care what others do around her. Although some women ask for a meal they very rarely tolerate it. Two slices of toast, with butter, jam, or honey served with tea or coffee is often plenty!

The nurse checks the woman's blood pressure and pulse and respiratory rates every 15 minutes. The temperature is checked hourly. The fundus of the uterus is checked to ensure that it is firm and well-contracted. The lochia or blood loss from the vagina is checked to be sure only a normal amount of blood loss occurs.

The woman now receives a full bed bath and pericare. At the end of one hour, provided all the vital signs are stable, the patient is taken to her room on the postpartum ward. Here, depending on how she feels, the new mother may rest and sleep for several hours, or she may continue to enjoy the company of her husband and baby.

Chapter 12
Psychoprophylaxis

Psychoprophylaxis means mind prevention or prevention of pain. It is a technique of prepared childbirth that is *family-unit oriented* involving mother and coach (the coach can be the husband, the woman's mother, or a friend). You are to experience pregnancy, labour, and delivery together in the most positive way, both playing an active role in the birth process.

Psychoprophylaxis is a structured but flexible technique that takes into consideration the needs of the couple. It offers you tools which are a set of predictable and adaptive behaviours in response to the contractions of labour.

Psychoprophylaxis is based on three principles: conditioning, discipline, and concentration. These three principles are described in the following paragraphs.

CONDITIONING

This principle is based on the Russian psychologist Pavlov's principle of conditioned response. Using Pavlov's principle, you learn through repetitions to respond to the stimulus of the contractions in a predictable way. That is, instead of tensing your body in response to the contractions you learn to remain calm and in control throughout. The tools or new behaviours you will learn are controlled relaxation and breathing techniques. This permits you to play an active role in your labour period. The coach's role is to supply verbal encouragement and other appropriate comfort measures.

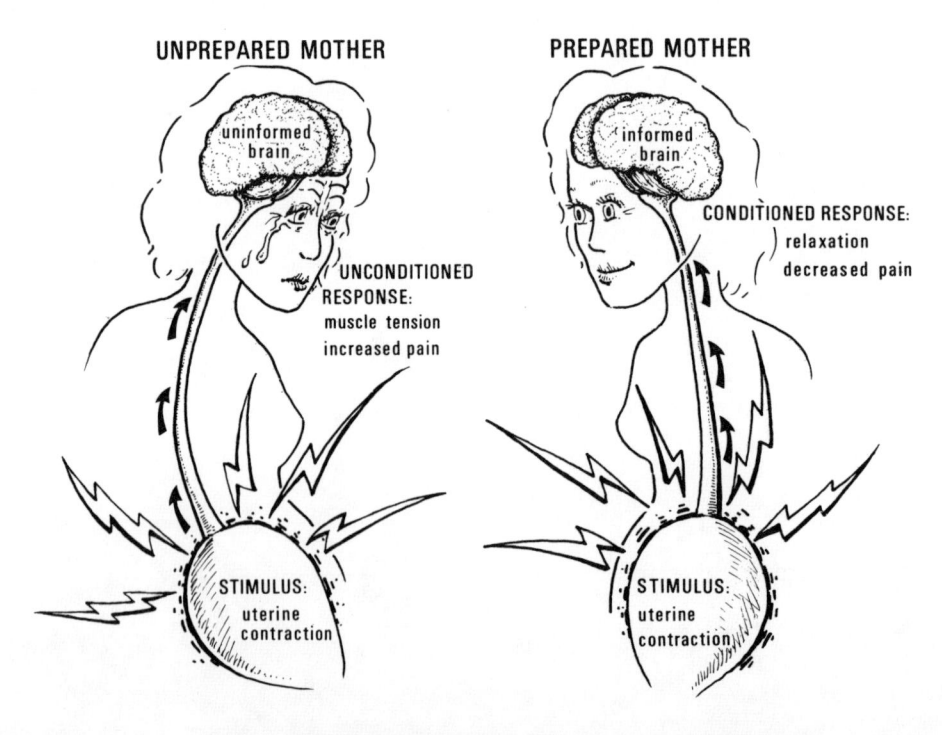

Figure 12.1. Conditioning: Prepared vs. Unprepared.

DISCIPLINE

During pregnancy you and your coach must practise the techniques taught in order for the conditioning process to occur, for only through repetition does a response become automatic. Take, for example, the driver of an automobile who no longer requires to analyze every step of driving his car. After months of repeating the same actions, it has become automatic.

CONCENTRATION

You learn to become oblivious to the activities around you so that you can truly concentrate on the techniques that you have practised. The focal point, which may be a picture or a chip on the ceiling paint, becomes the centre of your gaze during each contraction.

A woman who has been taught psychoprophylaxis will often require less medication (or no medication) compared to one with no training. Furthermore, you and your partner will be able to work more effectively with the rest of the obstetrical team. Finally, the success of this course is defined in terms of your satisfaction and enjoyable experience in the labour and delivery of your baby.

Chapter 13
Breathing Techniques for Labour

You must learn to respond to uterine contractions with a controlled type of breathing. That is, where active labour has progressed far enough for you to require support in order to stay calm, the start of a contraction should be a signal for you to start concentrating on controlled breathing and relaxation. It is this response to a contraction that should be automatic through your practice sessions. Instead of concentrating on the contractions of the uterus over which you have no control, you learn to concentrate on the muscles over which you do have control.

This concentration on controlled breathing and relaxation acts as a distraction and thereby lessens the sense of pain. Furthermore, correct breathing keeps a balanced amount of carbon dioxide and oxygen in the body. As you require more energy in the progression of labour, you will vary your breathing level accordingly from a slow deep chest breathing to a quicker more shallow type.

1. DCB deep chest breathing
2. MDCB modified deep chest breathing
3. Combined pattern MDCB—SCB—MDCB
4. SCB shallow chest breathing
5. SCB↑↓SCB accelerated, decelerated
6. SCB with puff blows

DCB and SCB are the basic breathing techniques; the remainder are modifications.

You will begin using the basic level when it is needed, starting only when walking or talking no longer appears to be comfortable. Thus, the levels of breathing do not coincide exactly with the stage of labour you may be in, since each woman will start utilizing the techniques at a different time. You will also use the progressive levels at different speeds. There are, however, some guidelines to follow.

Further on, are examples of the contractions in active labour. The curve represents only the approximate length of the contraction; the zigzag line represents the pattern of breathing you may be using.

Remember to begin and end each contraction with a deep cleansing breath, which is represented by the first and last zigzag in the diagram. This cleansing breath will also be a signal for the coach to time the contraction, or to offer support, verbal cues, or comfort measures. Remember also your focal point and the relaxation techniques as outlined.

Breathing Techniques for Labour 69

1. *DCB (Deep Chest Breathing)*

Inhale through the nose. Exhale through a relaxed mouth at the rate of eight breaths per minute (BPM).

Begin DCB in early labour when you feel the need for controlled breathing. Place your hands on your chest (beneath breast level) and feel your ribs expanding as you perform the DCB.

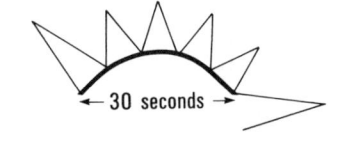

Figure 13.1.   DCB.

2. *MDCB (Modified Deep Chest Breathing)*

Same as DCB except more shallow and at the rate of 16 to 20 BPM.

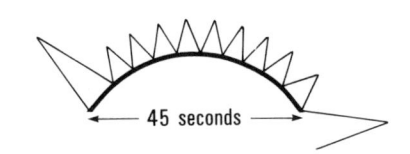

Figure 13.2.   MDCB.

3. *Combined Pattern*

Use MDCB as the contraction reaches a peak; use SCB (see pattern) as the contraction is peaking. Revert to MDCB as the contraction eases off.

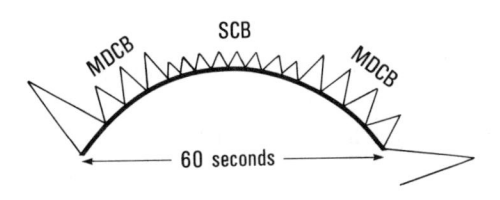

Figure 13.3.   Combined Pattern.

4. *SCB (Shallow Chest Breathing)*

Breathe in through the mouth. Breathe out through the mouth at the rate of 16 to 30 BPM. Breathing is light, effortless, and localized to the upper chest with minimal exertion of the lateral chest wall.

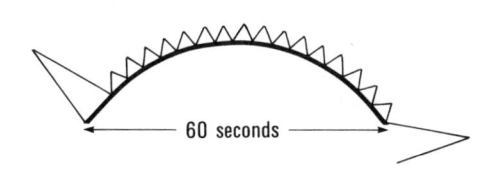

Figure 13.4.   SCB.

5. *SCB* ↑↓

Same as SCB except you will accelerate (breathing will become progressively more shallow and slightly quicker as the contraction intensifies). Decelerate breathing when the contraction eases off. Use with backache labour or very difficult contractions.

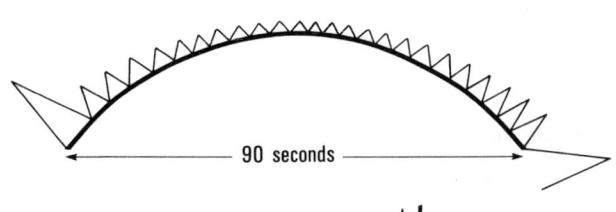

Figure 13.5.   SCB ↑↓.

6. *SCB With Puff Blows*

For every four SCB breaths there is one puff blow (i.e., expel all air from your lungs). The progression as the contractions become more difficult may be:

3 SCB to 1 puff blow
2 SCB to 1 puff blow
1 SCB to 1 puff blow

With an urge to push, you may do repeated puff blows until the urge has gone or until the cervix has fully dilated. Example of the breathing pattern in a contraction with an urge to push.

Use the above pattern in transition.

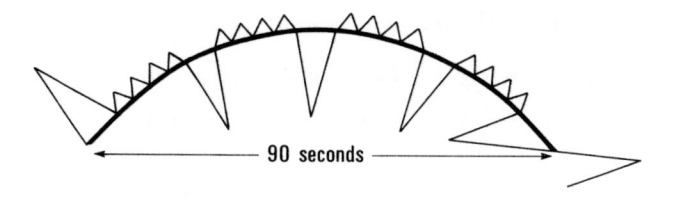

Figure 13.6. SCB With Puff Blows.

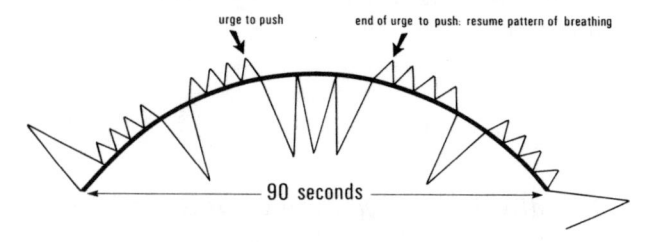

Figure 13.7. Urge to Push: Transitional Pattern.

When the cervix has dilated to 10 cm., it is time to start "bearing down" or pushing. The contractions are strong at this time, coupled with a tremendous desire to push. Before introducing the technique to follow during these contractions, it is important to point out that you should not practise "pushing" unless you are actually in labour.

1. Take two cleansing breaths quickly.

2. Inhale a third time and hold for ten seconds as you push or bear down through pursed lips slowly and steadily, in a forward direction (i.e., as if forcing to urinate). At the same time you are inhaling in preparation to push, your coach is helping you to assume the pushing position (you are then semi-reclined). If available, use the handle on either side of the table to help support yourself. Remember to relax your pelvic floor muscles as you are pushing.

3. Continue to bear down to the count of ten seconds. Then, blow out all the air. Take another deep breath in, hold your breath once again, and push to the count of ten seconds, through pursed lips slowly and steadily.

4. Repeat this pattern until the contraction is over, then lie back down with a deep cleansing breath. Relax until the next contraction.

You may be asked to stop pushing at some point when the baby's head is being born. In this instance you may use repeated puff blows.

PROGRESSION OF BREATHING PATTERN IN LABOUR

As labour progresses, the pattern of breathing becomes more shallow and quicker in order to cope with the increasing intensity of the contractions. As indicated earlier, only when you find that one

Breathing Techniques for Labour 71

level of breathing is ineffective would you begin using the next level. For instance, as the contractions become stronger, you will progress from DCB to MDCB, if you feel that DCB is no longer keeping you in control.

However, if you progress too soon with the breathing levels you will have no reserve for later labour. Also, if you breathe too quickly you may hyperventilate, that is, blow off too much CO_2, making the CO_2 blood level drop. Symptoms may include dizziness and blurring of vision. In such an instance, slow down your breathing, or hold your breath for a few seconds, or breathe into your cupped hands.

Try to remain at the lowest level of breathing for as long as you can. Remember also the few fundamental techniques given in each section of relaxation.

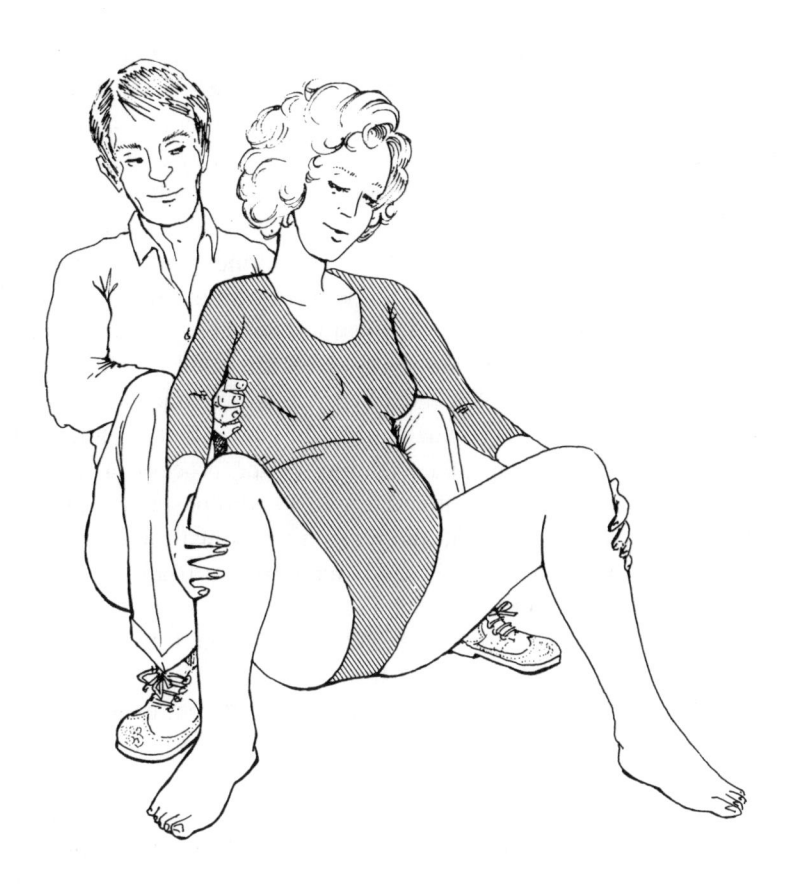

Figure 13.8. Semi-Reclining Pushing Position.
Your coach is helping you to assume the pushing position.

Chapter 14
Pain—Easing the Way

One truth we gain from living through the years,
Fear brings more pain than does the pain it fears.

John Golden

How painful is labour and what can be done to relieve it? It is very difficult to answer this question. Traditionally, childbirth has been seen as one of the greatest of all agonies and old wives' tales abound describing the dreadful sufferings that someone's mother, aunt, sister, or neighbour has undergone. However, there are many women who will assure that labour can be a relatively painless and exhilarating experience, while it may sometimes be a difficult and trying ordeal.

To the woman who has some understanding of the childbirth process, who has trust in her obstetrician, plus support and understanding from her partner, the experience of having a baby can be one of great joy and fulfillment. These are the women who use psychoprophylaxis or the "unmedicated childbirth" method with great success. For most women, the experience will fall somewhere between these extremes; some labours are more exhausting and painful, but feelings of discomfort and pain vary so much that every labour must be treated as a unique experience.

There are many reasons for these differences. In labour there is a fear of the unknown, thus it follows that the couple who have an understanding of the process of labour and delivery are less likely to experience fear. It was Dr. Grantley Dick Read who postulated that, "Fear increases tension which in turn further increases fear. Fear and tension mean that the mother's body pulls against the action of the muscles of the birth canal. If she is anxious and frightened her body will be tense and relaxation will be difficult. Labour is the natural culmination of pregnancy and simply means hard work. Throughout the three stages of labour the uterus or womb (the hollow muscular organ in which your baby lives for the first nine months of his life) contracts with very powerful muscular movements interpreted by most women as painful. These very powerful contractions are needed firstly to aid in opening up the cervix wide enough to allow passage of your baby's head into the vagina and secondly to help in pushing your baby down through the birth canal and out into the world."

With this pain, fear increases, making the tension (tightness) greater, thereby producing more pain, so that a vicious circle of pain and tension is established. Furthermore, labour is a very tiring process. In order to conserve energy, you must work with your body, not against it. It has been said many times that fatigue is the greatest enemy of the labouring woman.

The process of giving birth is unique, a highly subjective experience. Thus cultural background plays an important role. Different social groups have specific characteristics and expectations of what constitutes "normal" behaviour. One group may feel that a woman who makes a lot of noise during labour is behaving badly while others find a display of noise and suffering not only acceptable but necessary. An important point about labour must be made here; regardless of preparation and training, there may be times during labour and delivery when some form of pain-relieving medication may be advised by your obstetrician. If this happens, it should not be viewed as a failure on your part nor a waste of the effort that you have put into learning. It simply means that every birth is different and, because all human beings are individuals, reactions will vary.

Whatever the cause and/or degree of pain, no caring doctor or nurse wants to see a woman in labour suffer unnecessarily. They want to relieve her discomfort while making sure her baby is in good health. However, this creates a problem; drugs given to relieve pain can pass from the placenta (afterbirth) to the baby, and too much medication can result in a drugged baby. The hard work and trauma of labour and birth are enough for the newborn; he does not need the added strain of medication in his small body. This is the reason that drugs are so carefully chosen and meticulously controlled.

The choice of pain-relieving medication should be decided mutually by you, your obstetrician, and the anesthesiologist. A variety of methods are available today and have proven to be safe and effective for you and your baby. These types of anesthesia include sedatives, narcotics, local anesthesia, regional anesthesia, epidural anesthesia, and inhalation analgesia (Entonox).

SEDATIVES

Sedatives are occasionally used in very early labour to promote sleep. If, for example, you become fatigued due to irregular and ineffective contractions and you are *not* established in labour, your obstetrician may order a sedative. This will help you to obtain a few hours of sleep in order to reduce your fatigue before going into regular (established) labour.

NARCOTICS

Morphine and Demerol (Pethidine, Meperdine) have been used in obstetrics for many years, but are not commonly used these days because of potential danger to the unborn child; i.e., they reduce the baby's respiratory rate if given close to the time of birth.

LOCAL ANESTHESIA

Infiltration of the Perineum

This is the direct injection of an anesthetic agent such as xylocaine into the area of discomfort (similar to the dentist freezing your gum prior to dental work). Your perineal area will be infiltrated with this pain-killing drug either just before the episiotomy is performed or when it is being sutured following delivery of your baby. You will be in the delivery position, and usually you will be only minimally aware of the injection as your tissues are very distended (the head of the baby "thins out" the perineum and also exerts direct pressure on the nerves of this area).

If you need a local anesthetic, this will be performed by your obstetrician. (It will relieve pain only in the perineal area).

REGIONAL ANESTHESIA

Regional anesthetics are injections into and/or around the sympathetic nerve pathways. They block impulses and so numb the area and reduce painful sensations.

PARACERVICAL BLOCK

Paracervical block may be administered in the first stage of labour, e.g., at 5 to 6 cm. It blocks the sensation of nerves supplying the uterus.

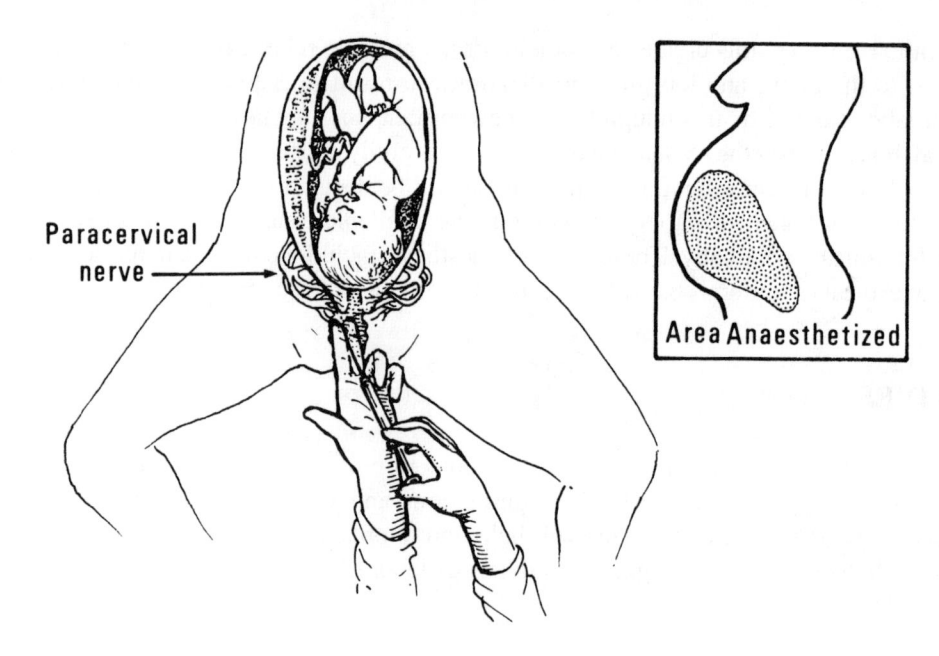

Figure 14.1. Paracervical Nerve Block.

PUDENDAL BLOCK

Pudendal block is used to relieve pain in the vaginal area and perineal area for the second stage of labour and delivery.

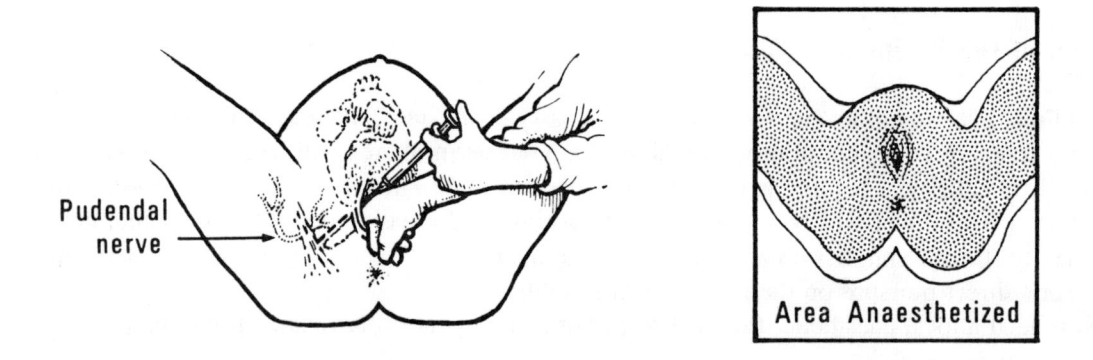

Figure 14.2. Pudendal Nerve Block.

EPIDURAL ANESTHESIA

This is a regional nerve blockage of the nerve roots in the epidural space, which is between the spinal dura and the vertebral bone (see diagram). Epidural anesthesia involves the passage of a small flexible polyethylene (plastic) catheter into your lower back. The anesthetist injects an anesthetic medication, e.g. xylocaine, through the catheter to dull the pain of your contractions. In most cases epidural anesthesia provides excellent pain relief, though feelings of pressure and/or mild discomfort may remain.

Pain—Easing the Way

Epidural anesthesia may be started any time during labour but is usually not begun until your contractions are strong and regular, i.e., when labour is well established with a cervical dilatation of 4 cm. If your epidural is administered before you are in active labour it may slow down or even stop your labour. In certain conditions, epidural anesthesia may not be advisable. These are:

1. Antepartum hemorrhage, e.g. placenta previa.

2. Severe, chronic back pain, e.g. sciatica, disc disease, and previous back surgery.

3. Neurological disease, e.g. multiple sclerosis.

4. Abnormal bleeding tendencies.

It is necessary that you inform your anesthetist of any of the above problems, any medications that you are taking, and any allergic reactions or adverse effects you may have had from previous surgery and/or anesthesia.

Insertion of the epidural catheter will be done by your anesthetist. Your nurse will help to position you either lying on your side or sitting up. It is very important that you move as little as possible while the procedure is being performed. When you are having a contraction, the anesthetist will stop until this has finished. Various sensations may be experienced during the epidural. One of these is an "electric shock," or tingling in your back and legs. This is an uncomfortable rather than a painful sensation. Once the catheter is inserted, the medication will be injected through it and you may notice some shivering, heaviness, or numbness in your legs; this is quite normal.

During this period your blood pressure and the baby's heart rate are carefully monitored. You must lie on your side as this is anatomically advantageous for your baby and your blood pressure. (The reason for this is known medically as "supine hypotension," which simply means that the pressure

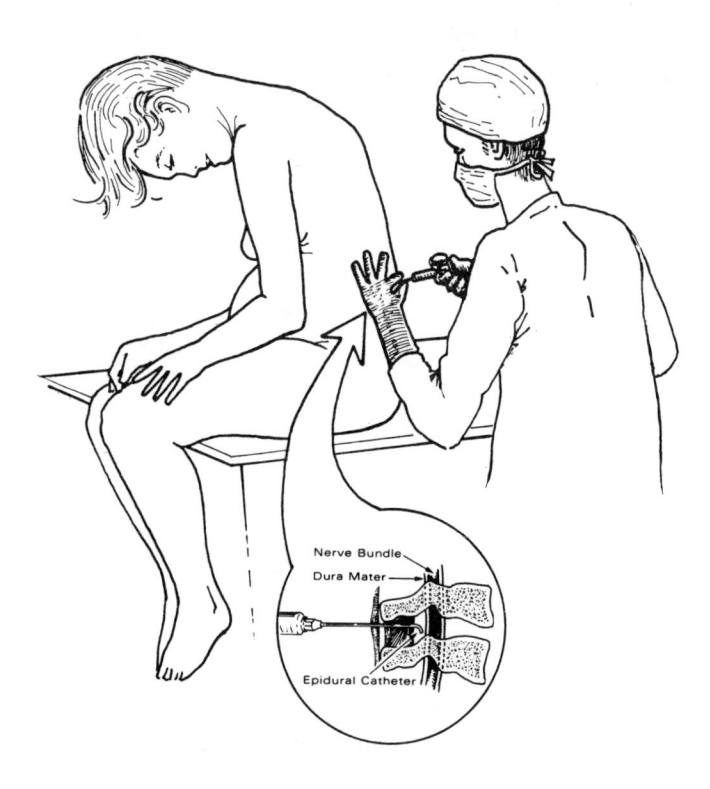

Figure 14.3. Epidural Anesthesia.

of the heavy uterus when you are lying flat on your back can restrict the flow of blood to major blood vessels.) Every one to three hours, repeated injections of the medication will be made through the catheter in order to provide continuous pain relief. This is called the "topping up" procedure.

As labour progresses and the second stage is reached, you will be moved from a lying to a sitting position so that gravity can aid the spread of the medication down the epidural space to reach and bathe the nerve endings that supply the vagina and the lower part of the birth canal. Because the epidural removes varying degrees of sensation, your partner and/or nurse will assist you in pushing effectively in the second stage.

Soon after your baby is delivered, the anesthetist will remove the epidural catheter from your back. Initially your legs will feel heavy but this sensation will eventually disappear in a few hours. You will then be allowed up if you wish, though assistance from a nurse is recommended for your first trip to the bathroom.

INHALATION ANALGESIA (ENTONOX)

Inhalation analgesia (if available in your hospital) is usually offered in the advance stage of labour.

Entonox is a mixture of 50% nitrous oxide and 50% oxygen. It is self-administered by the patient using a hand-held face mask with a valve and a cylinder tubing (see diagram).

Your anesthetist will show you how to use the mask. In order to obtain full effect of the gas, you should breathe deeply through the mask during your contractions. With this form of analgesia, you have complete control over the amount of anesthesia you receive.

The best solution is to realize right from the start that the decision on medication is yours.

If your contractions are too uncomfortable, ask for help; likewise, if you are offered pain relief and you feel that the pain is still quite bearable, then you are completely within your rights to refuse.

Whatever methods are used to alleviate the pain of childbirth, expectant parents are naturally apprehensive. The aim of childbirth education preparation is to try to overcome this anxiety. By providing knowledge to increase understanding and confidence, we can help you to achieve that sense of satisfaction and happiness that accompanies bringing a new life into the world.

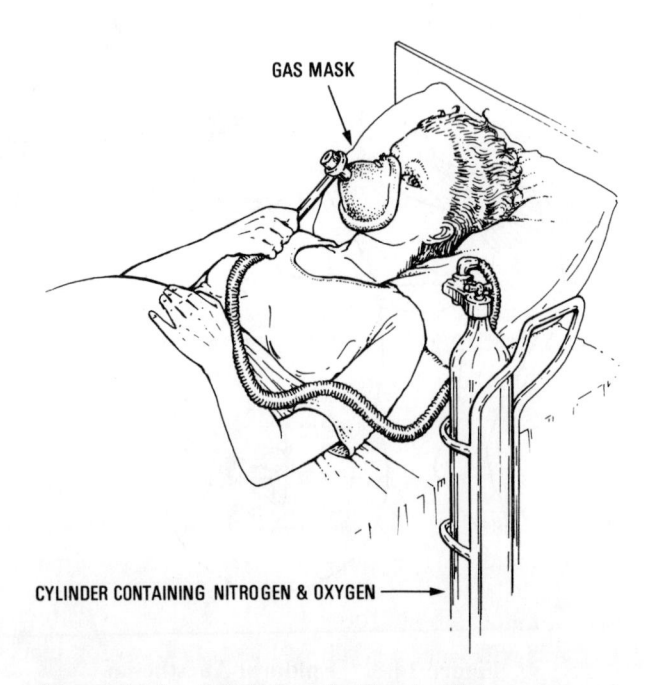

Figure 14.4. Inhalation Analgesia (Entonox).

Chapter 15
Coach's Reminder Sheet

HOW TO HELP YOUR PARTNER DURING LABOUR

Early Labour

1. Be calm and have confidence in yourself. Remember your presence and companionship are most important contributions. You have a unique emotional tie with your partner.

2. If the contractions begin at night, and they are mild, urge your partner to get more sleep. If contractions start during the daytime, help her pass the time by reading, playing cards, watching television, talking, walking, etc.

3. Do not force her to go to bed if she does not wish. Most women prefer sitting in a comfortable chair with head, arms, and legs supported, or walking about for brief periods, pausing momentarily to support the body and relax with the contractions. Time contractions, duration and frequency.

4. Your partner should not start her controlled breathing until she feels the need (when she can no longer walk or talk comfortably during a contraction). When she does, her breathing should be slow and even. At this stage of her labour, she will probably be in control of herself, and her breathing, and a few words of praise and reassurance from you is all that is needed. Eating and drinking anything but clear fluids should be avoided when contractions have begun.

5. Call the admitting office before going to the hospital. If your partner cannot contact her doctor and needs advice, then phone directly to the labour room.

6. *The trip to the hospital*: You should know the route, the approximate time it will take, and the correct entrance to the hospital in advance. Don't let the gas tank get down to empty during the last few weeks of the pregnancy. *Drive carefully*, avoiding sudden stops and rapid turns. There's plenty of time; remind your partner to relax and breathe slowly and rhythmically with contractions. Have a practice run. Do not bring any valuables or a lot of money. Leave the suitcase in the car. Do bring your Lamaze Goodie Bag (containing talcum powder, pencil and writing paper, and a tennis ball) and a light lunch for dad, but remember that you are responsible for your goodie bag when you leave the labour room. Things required in the labour room are: slippers, toilet bag with toothbrush and chapstick, etc., book or magazine, sanitary belt, and at least two pillows.

7. On arrival at the hospital, follow instructions for completing admission, accompany your wife to the labour and delivery area, if in advanced labour.

8. While you are in the labour room with your partner, street clothes have to be removed and you will wear a scrub suit and shoe covers; place your street clothes

in the locker provided for your partner for her clothes, unless instructed otherwise. When you want to call for a nurse, use the call system provided in the labour room. If you take a break, go to the father's waiting room, *do not wander around the labour and delivery area*. Do not smoke or eat in the labour room. The operating room is off limits, and so is the information board with information on all patients in the labour room. If your partner is having a cesarean and you are given permission to be present by your doctor, then you are allowed in the operating room.

9. Discourage all phone calls from relatives during labour. If you leave the labour room, you have to change completely. Bring money for phone calls, and for your locker.

Active Labour

1. Contractions are definitely stronger, closer, and more determined or more predictable; i.e., longer, stronger, and more frequent. Your partner no longer wants to chat but becomes quiet and preoccupied with her labour. Do not disturb her or distract her during contractions with idle talk; the contractions demand her deep concentration. The coach must be involved with the contractions by giving verbal cues and encouraging her as needed. It sometimes helps to do actual breathing exercises with your partner if she forgets the correct technique.

2. *A quiet, subdued environment will aid her ability to relax.* Avoid bright lights shining in her eyes, excessive chatter, and movements in the room.

3. *Position of your partner is important to her physical comfort and ability to relax.* In the back relaxation position, the head of the bed should be elevated about 45 degrees and the knees should be flexed slightly with an additional pillow under her knees (contour chair-like position). In the side relaxation position, the bed should be flat with your partner on her side. The upper leg is bent forward, supported on a pillow, another pillow being under the head. Urge her to change positions often and help her to move, elevate, or lower the bed and rearrange pillows.

4. *"Backache Labour"*: Often due to occiput posterior presentation (baby's head pressing against mother's back); can be relieved by:

    a. Firm constant pressure of coach's fists against woman's sacrum.

    b. Frequent changes in position.

    c. Pelvic rocking in sidelying position.

    d. Using the technique of S.C.B., at accelerated-decelerated rate; encouraging partner to void hourly.

    The S.C.B. technique is very tiring and should be used only when absolutely necessary or if the contractions are very, very difficult.

5. *Women in labour appreciate gestures of comfort:* Touching, cool, wet washcloth to wipe her face and neck; cracked ice, lemon or lime lollipop, to moisten her dry mouth; chapstick, hard candy (all of which are brought in your Lamaze Goodie Bag).

6. *Offer frequent words of encouragement:* Such words as, "You're doing nicely," "Wonderful," "Keep it up," do not come often enough. The use of positive sugges-

tions such as "Your contraction is at its peak and will soon let up" may help. It may also help to mark off 15-second time intervals for her.

7. *Help her with her controlled breathing:* Remember this is her best tool to aid her relaxation and the diversion of her attention off uterine contractions. Remind her to concentrate on her focal point, cleansing breath before and after each contraction, offer effleurage as long as the abdomen is not too sensitive. She should use the deep chest breathing as long as possible, changing to modified deep chest breathing, to combined pattern as necessary.

8. At times you might feel frustrated and lost, standing by, feeling you're not doing or offering much, especially if your partner has difficulty controlling her contractions. *Always remember your presence is the most welcome emotional and physical support for her.*

9. Feel free to enquire regarding cervical dilatation following each pelvic examination. It is reasonable to request one or two pelvic examinations only during labour.

Transition (8 to 10 centimeters) is the Most Demanding Period of Labour

The contractions are long, strong, and one after another. She may feel overwhelmed, unable to go on. She will be irritable, discouraged, and may momentarily panic. She will need your help now more than at any other time. She will need firm directions as to what to do with each contraction.

1. Discontinue effleurage because the abdomen is too sensitive.

2. Remind her that this period is short, and relief will come with the second stage; think only of one contraction at a time and that there is a rest period after each contraction. Remind her that soon the baby will be born.

3. If she has medication she may doze between contractions and be confused when she wakes. Speak to her when the contraction starts and tell her to keep her eyes open and focus her attention on whomever is guiding her.

4. If she panics and momentarily loses control, speak to her in a firmer voice saying "breathe in and out, keep it up and keep it even," etc., until the contraction is over. Breathe with her to keep her going.

5. If she has increasing low backache, the firm steady pressure of the heel of your hand during the contraction may help to ease the discomfort or may aggravate it in some cases. Remind her that this will pass and the baby will be born. Do not fuss too much; ask questions that can be answered yes or no; give moral support.

6. The catch in her breathing, or a sensation that she cannot breathe, with the urge to move her bowels, signals the onset of the second stage (expulsive stage). Urge her to continue shallow chest breathing with "puff blow" at rhythmic intervals. When the urge to push occurs do "repeated blows" until the urge has stopped. Make sure the nurses and doctors know of her desire to push. Remind her to continue her breathing and puff blow to prevent pushing until she is told to go ahead.

Second Stage

The expulsive or pushing stage will bring mixed feelings of surprise and joy: surprise by the strange and indescribable power, and joy because it signals anticipation of birth. She needs to be reassured that the sensations are normal and pushing brings relief. She will need direct guidance as to what to do.

1. When the doctor or nurse gives her the "go ahead" to push, encourage her to take two cleansing breaths. Support her in semi-reclined position (i.e., 45 degrees), tell her to take a third deep breath, hold it and bear down while focusing between her knees. Count aloud to ten or as needed while she continues to bear down. Then she should breathe out, quickly take in another breath and continue pushing through the count of ten or as needed. Continue in the same fashion until the end of the contraction. Let her lie back and finish with a cleansing breath.

2. Informing her of her progress encourages her to push and work harder.

3. In the delivery room, you will be at your partner's shoulder or head. Keep her informed of what is happening and repeat the doctor's instructions to her if necessary. Your voice is familiar and she will respond to it readily. If she wishes to watch the birth in the mirror, remind her to keep her eyes open. You may watch the birth of the baby in the mirror, *but please do not move around the room.*

4. Encourage your partner to use deep chest breathing when the doctor says not to push during delivery.

5. Discuss with your doctor whether photos can be taken in delivery room or operating room.

After Delivery

1. Be sure to praise your partner's hard work.

2. From the delivery room your partner and baby will go back to the recovery area (labour room, recovery room), for a while, until the bed is ready in the postpartum area.

3. You and your partner will be together with your baby during the recovery period for approximately 10 to 20 minutes.

4. You may hold and touch your baby.

5. Ask the nurse if your partner wishes to breastfeed or hold the baby right away on the delivery room table, or if you want to hold the baby in the delivery room.

6. Do not forget your money for your phone calls.

7. Follow instructions for removal of your delivery room clothes.

8. You can accompany your partner to the postpartum area or recovery room following a cesarean birth. You may also go to the nursery with your baby.

Good Luck!

Chapter 16
Guidelines to Couples Participating in Labour

The tables in this chapter present useful guidelines to couples participating in labour. Table 16.1 summarizes "what is happening" in the weeks and days preceding labour, and offers suggestions to help both the expectant mother and the coach. Table 16.2 lists physical and emotional changes that characterize the various stages of labour, and includes suggestions for the mother and the coach at each stage. Tables 16.3 and 16.4 describe steps you may take in the event of hyperventilation or back labour. Of course, every birth is unique, and your experience may differ in some ways from the general description given here.

Table 16.1. Prelude to Labour

What is Happening	Helping Yourself	Coaching and Support
Lightening: (Descent of the presenting part, usually the head, into the pelvis) 2–4 weeks before first baby comes.	Simplify housekeeping. Have hospital suitcase packed. Conserve energy.	Share her excitement and happiness about the coming event.
Braxton-Hicks Contractions (intermittent, painless uterine contractions present throughout pregnancy) may increase.	Try different relaxation positions.	
Increased vaginal discharge.	Organize a tour of the hospital and have your registration completed.	
Baby less active.		
Excitement about labour may make sleeping difficult.		
Spurt of energy (1–2 days before labour).		
Mucus plug "show" (vaginal discharge with a pink or red tinge) days to weeks prior to labour.		

Table 16.2. Stages of Labour

Stage	Characterized By	Emotional Reactions	Coaching and Support
ONSET OF LABOUR Do not go to the hospital too soon.	You may notice any one of a combination of regular contractions (felt as backache, pelvic pressure, gas, menstrual cramps, etc.) "Show." Leaking of Fluid.	You may feel excited and relieved that labour has begun, and yet somewhat apprehensive. Keep up your regular activities. Time contractions with finger tips on the abdomen. Note the duration of each contraction as well as the rest period between each. (If partner is not home.) Review relaxation techniques.	Be calm and have confidence in yourself. Time contractions, duration and frequency. A few words of praise and reassurance from you are all that is needed.
EARLY PHASE OF 1ST STAGE Effacement—Cervix thinning out. Early Dilatation—Cervix beginning to open. *0–4 cm.* Longer in comparison to other phases.	*CONTRACTIONS:* Every 5–30 minutes lasting 30–45 sec. Mild and irregular, then becoming stronger and regular. May be felt as: Menstrual cramps, gas, headache, pelvic pressure, or tightening low down in area of pubic bone. *SHOW:* None, or slightly pinkish mucus discharge. *MEMBRANES:* May rupture up to 24 hours before labour, or at any time during labour; or may be ruptured by doctor. After rupture, fluid may gush or trickle from vagina.	Excited and relieved. Some apprehension. Sociable and talkative between contractions. Slight discomfort with contractions. Air of anticipation. Impatient and eager for progress. Do not eat or drink. Avoid fatigue. *Night:* Sleep or rest. *Day:* Light housework, T.V., reading, cards, walking, etc. Start slow deep chest breathing (5–8 min.) with contractions only when necessary. Maintain relaxation. It is important to keep your energy.	Encourage diversional activity. Time the frequency and duration of contractions periodically. Support and encouragement. Check for relaxation. Give back rub if needed.

Table 16.2.—*Continued.*

Stage	Characterized By	Emotional Reactions	Coaching and Support
MIDDLE PHASE OF 1ST STAGE Effacement should be complete. *4–8 cm.* Usually shorter than the early phase.	CONTRACTIONS: Every 3–5 minutes lasting 40–60 sec., businesslike, more regular, becoming closer, markedly stronger and of longer duration. Uncomfortable. SHOW: Increased bloody show. PROGRESSION OF BREATHING TECHNIQUES: Modified Deep Chest Breathing. Combined pattern. M.D.C.B., Shallow Chest Breathing, M.D.C.B. FOR VERY DIFFICULT CONTRACTIONS OR BACKACHE LABOUR S.C.B. at accelerated-decelerated rate. Do not overbreathe.	Increasingly serious, quieter, preoccupied with self and labour. Increasingly dependent and needs quiet companionship. May worry about ability to see labour through. Works hard during contractions and prefers not to talk or be distracted. Relaxation difficult.	Needs frequent reassurance, encouragement, coaching, and continuous companionship. Needs relaxed quiet environment. Avoid bright lights shining in her eyes, and excessive chatter. Accept her irritability. REMIND HER TO: *Concentrate on a focal point:* Relax body, jaw, perineum, and limbs. Take a cleansing breath before and after every contraction. Relax between contractions and concentrate on one contraction at a time. Void and change position frequently. Use massaging (effleurage) or straightening to relax limbs and relieve tension over the abdomen. FOR BACKACHE LABOUR: Apply counter pressure to sacrum with fist or heel of your hand, or tennis balls. Frequent changes in position. Pelvic rocking in sidelying position. Wipe her forehead, face, and neck with a cool cloth if necessary, moisten lips from time to time.

Table 16.2.—*Continued.*

Stage	Characterized By	Emotional Reactions	Coaching and Support
TRANSITION PHASE OF 1ST STAGE *8–10 cms.* Very intensive but shortest stage. Usually lasts from 10–20 contractions.	CONTRACTIONS: Every 2–3 min. lasting 60–90 sec.—very strong (seems continuous to patient). *SHOW:* Heavy and dark. May have—hiccups, nausea and vomiting, amnesia between contractions, leg cramps, trembling of extremities, backache, perspiration on forehead and around eyes, cheeks may appear flushed, may feel hot or cold, restless, relaxation is very difficult, sleepy and drowsy between contractions, rectal pressure may cause desire to bear down (urge to push). *BREATHING TECHNIQUES* S.C.B. with rhythmic "Puff—Blow" *FOR URGE TO PUSH:* Repeated "Blows"	Irritable, sensitive, and short-tempered, cannot communicate verbally, overwhelmed and wants to give up. Bewildered, frustrated and temporarily discouraged, exhausted. *CANNOT BEAR TO BE LEFT ALONE* Considerable difficulty concentrating and relaxing during and between contractions. May be surprised, overwhelmed, or even frightened at irresistible urge to push.	*NEVER LEAVE HER ALONE* *Needs constant encouragement, coaching, and reassurance* of normality of sensations and progress. Coach's face becomes focal point. Discontinue stroking abdomen. Needs firm positive guidance, continuous low key verbal coaching and breathing with her through each contraction often helps. *REMIND HER:* That phase is short and pushing will feel better; birth is imminent. Remind her to change position—to sit up with back supported, knees spread apart, heels together—to keep eyes open and concentrate—to have bladder empty—to relax pelvic floor. *OFFER:* Back pressure—if necessary, ice chips, wet cloth, constant coaching and praise. *NOTIFY STAFF OF HER DESIRE TO PUSH.*

Guidelines to Couples

Table 16.2.—*Continued.*

Stage	Characterized By	Emotional Reactions	Coaching and Support
SECOND STAGE THE EXPULSIVE STAGE *Pushing and Delivery* Total time of second stage: anywhere from 5 to 60 or more minutes.	CONTRACTIONS: Change in character, remaining very strong but slightly further apart. Continuing strong contractions pushing baby down against pelvic floor and causing stretching, perhaps burning sensation. Baby's head seen (vaginal opening). As doctor slowly delivers head, there may be strong desire to push. Shoulders are born one at a time. Relief is experienced as birth of baby is completed. The doctor may do an episiotomy (to facilitate delivery of baby).	Surprised and even overwhelmed or frightened by pushing sensation. *Very* tired but a revival of determination and burst of energy. Pressure on rectum may cause anxiety and hesitation to push. Tremendous effort may produce distorted facial expression and grunting on inhalation. Drowsy and peaceful between contractions. Self concern indifferent to surroundings, uninhibited, excited, absorbed in her own job, impatient for progress. Mental alertness and excitement replaces drowsiness and discouragement. Interest shifts to baby as birth occurs.	Needs coaching with each contraction. May "forget" how to push. Suggest she directs pushing toward one spot such as vagina and think "down and out." Have mirror adjusted if desired. *REMIND HER TO:* Take two cleansing breaths, then take a third breath and hold it while bearing down. Exhale through pursed lips, slowly and steadily. Back and shoulders rounded in a "C" curve. Pull upon the handles and keep the pelvis flat on bed or table from waist down. Relax pelvic floor. Coach provides support for shoulders during each push. Look in the mirror. For optimum efficiency 2–3 long pushes until the end of contraction. Take a cleansing breath after each contraction and relax. Tell her when the head is visible and describe progress. Praise her accomplishment.

Table 16.2.—*Continued.*

Stage	Characterized By	Emotional Reactions	Coaching and Support
THIRD STAGE Placental separation and expulsion. Very brief stage, often unnoticed by mother. Anywhere from 5 to 20 minutes, or more.	CONTRACTIONS: Temporarily cease after birth and may resume. Uterus rises in abdomen and takes globular shape (grapefruit size). Umbilical cord lengthens. Uterus contracts to expel placenta. Gush of blood may precede or accompany expulsion of placenta. Doctor or nurse may push on abdomen to aid expulsion. Oxytocin injection to contract uterus. Episiotomy repaired with local anesthetic.	Euphoria; pure ecstasy is common, relief, gratitude, disbelief, wonder, joy, excitement. Exhausted, but often too ecstatic to notice fatigue. Pride and fulfillment. May be annoyed when contractions resume. Ravenously hungry and thirsty. Delighted with flat abdomen. Focus on baby and seeks reassurance that baby is normal. May be sleepy when excitement subsides or so excited she is unable to sleep. Often unaware of placental expulsion or episiotomy repaired.	Join in mother's enthusiasm and wonder. Sit down and enjoy your baby together. Praise mother's accomplishment. Remind her that suctioning of baby, heated crib, etc., are routine procedures. Ask permission for mother to breastfeed baby if she desires. Hold baby.

Table 16.3. Hyperventilation

Rapid Deep Breathing in which Too Much Carbon Dioxide is Exhaled

Preventative Measures	Signs	Corrective Measures
1. Breathe at the slowest rate possible. 2. Concentrate on focal point.	1. Blurring of vision. 2. Light-headedness and 3. Tingling of hands and feet, progressing to cramps and muscle spasms in hands.	1. Slow down breathing. 2. Breathe into your hands. 3. Breathe into a small paper bag. 4. Hold your breath for a few seconds before inhaling.

Table 16.4. Suggestions for Relief of "Back Labour"

It is very important to concentrate on consciously relaxing your lower buttocks and thighs, not only during a contraction, but also between contractions.

Position	Relief Measures
1. Lie on your side, knees bent, with top leg supported by a pillow and drawn up slightly higher than the leg.	1. Apply firm pressure to lower back—partner may use palm of hand or fist. You may lie on your own fists—especially during a pelvic exam. Use tennis balls.
2. Sit up and lean forward supporting your weight over a pillow or pillows or dangle your feet over side of the bed and rest your arms on a bed table.	2. Do pelvic rocking in side lying.
	3. Back rub may help. Use talcum powder to help avoid friction on the skin.
3. You may be advised to push on your side rather than lying on your back if the baby is posterior.	4. Apply a warm, moist wash cloth to lower back.
	5. Deep massage starting with hard pressure at base of tailbone and working fingers up between buttocks, radiating out over lower back.
	6. Light massage of inner thighs and groin may help relaxation of pelvic and buttock area.

Chapter 17
Induction of Labour And Other Forms of Medical Intervention

An induction is done for two reasons: to prevent ill-health in the mother; and to preserve the life of the fetus (baby). Careful observation of the fetal heart, contractions, maternal pulse rate, and blood pressure must be recorded prior to starting the induction and will be monitored throughout the course of labour.

Induction of labour is carried out when there are significant indications to do so. Here are some obstetrical and medical indications.

INDICATIONS FOR INDUCTION OF LABOUR

Obstetrical	Medical	Poor Obstetrical History
Postmaturity (41 to 42 weeks)	Diabetes Mellitus	*For example:*
Pre-eclampsia (hypertension with proteinuria or edema or both)	Cardiac disease	infertility
Prolonged rupture of membranes	Asthmatic and epileptic patients	miscarriages
Rhesus incompatibility	Hypertension	previous complicated birth
Cephalo-pelvic disproportion (the size of the fetal head is large in relation to the maternal pelvis)	Other severe illnesses	
Multiple pregnancy (twins)		
Ante-partum hemorrhage		

The doctor usually explains the procedure to the patient in advance and arranges for her admission to the hospital. It is necessary to fast from midnight of the previous day. In the labour and delivery unit, the pubic hair is shaved (not always), and an enema is given if needed.

There are two methods of induction, medical and surgical. Sometimes the two methods are combined.

Surgical induction is done under the most sterile conditions. A vaginal examination is made by the doctor and the membranes are artificially ruptured with a small hook. This is not usually a painful procedure, but some women may find it uncomfortable. This can only be done if the cervix is dilating and the presenting part may be reached by the examining finger.

Medical induction involves the giving of medication, i.e., syntocinon (oxytocin), via an intravenous infusion to initiate and encourage labour.

Usually, if all is favourable, after six hours of syntocinon (oxytocin) therapy, most patients respond and would either be in the active phase of labour or be actually delivered. Some women claim that contractions start more abruptly than when one experiences the spontaneous onset of labour. When labour is induced, breathing techniques are often required from the outset of labour and perhaps there is a need for greater concentration. However, the procedure is safe and worthwhile when ordered by the doctor and good nursing and medical supervision is enforced. The fetal heart and contractions are monitored continuously.

The syntocinon (oxytocin) infusion is often continued after the birth and will be discontinued within *six* hours (on an average) provided the vital signs of the mother are normal, the fundus of the uterus is well contracted, and the urinary output is satisfactory.

FORCEPS DELIVERY

A forceps delivery may be necessary to provide for the safe delivery of your child. The doctor is the one who makes the decision to use forceps. You should know why the application of forceps is required.

Certain conditions must be present to allow a forceps delivery:

1. The cervix must be fully dilated.
2. The presenting part should be vertex (head).
3. The membranes have ruptured.
4. There is no disproportion between baby's head and mother's pelvis.
5. An episiotomy is made after freezing the perineal tissue with local anesthesia; a pudendal block is done; or if the patient is having continuous epidural anesthesia.

The obstetrical forceps are carefully designed to protect the fetal head and mother's birth canal.

A low forceps delivery is carried out when the largest presenting diameter is below the level of the ischial spines and the head is distending the perineum. The commonest indications are:

1. Rigid perineum.
2. Physical or emotional fatigue in mother.
3. Fetal distress.
4. Prematurity.
5. The after-coming head of a breech.

A mid-forceps delivery is done when the fetal head is engaged but the presenting part is at the level of the ischial spines. The indications are:

1. Deep transverse arrest causing delay in the second stage of labour.
2. Posterior positions of the vertex.

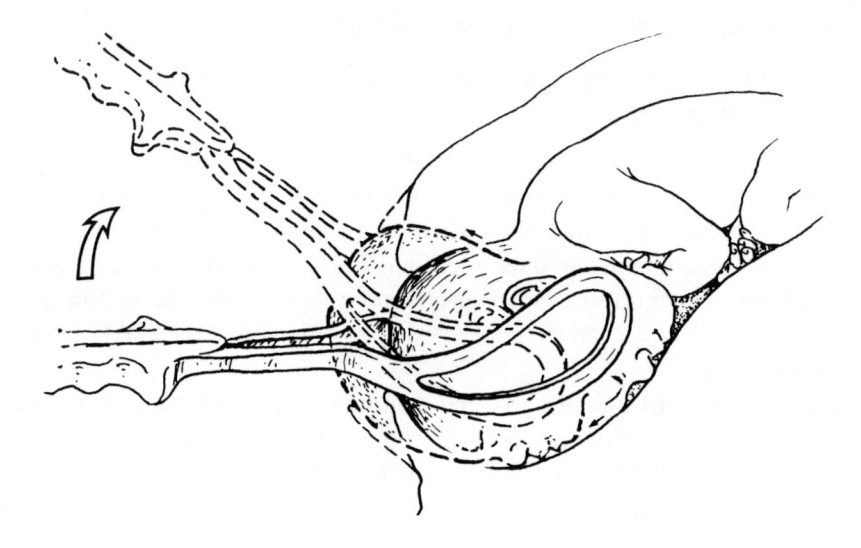

Figure 17.1. Forceps.

The situations above not only give rise to delay in the second stage but also to:

3. Fetal distress.

When there are maternal complications such as cardiac disease, pre-eclampsia, a forceps delivery may sometimes be required. The patient is usually placed in the delivery position, with the use of padded stirrups during the delivery.

EPISIOTOMY

An episiotomy is done to increase the vaginal opening during birth. This may be premeditated or decided upon during the actual delivery.

Local anesthesia is given to infiltrate the perineum, and a clean cut is made in the perineal tissue to facilitate the delivery of the baby. A sterile scissor is used by the doctor. The direction of the cut is made from the lower midline of the vagina towards the anus (median) for one to one and one-quarter inches or to one side at an angle of 45 degrees (medio-lateral). *Indications for an episiotomy are as follows:*

Premeditated

1. Cephalo-pelvic disproportion due to a large baby, the diameter of the head being greater than the essential diameters of the pelvis.
2. Multiple birth.
3. Prematurity.
4. Breech presentation.
5. Previous tear or episiotomy.
6. Snugness for partner.

Induction of Labour/Medical Intervention 91

medio-lateral   median
INCISION TYPES

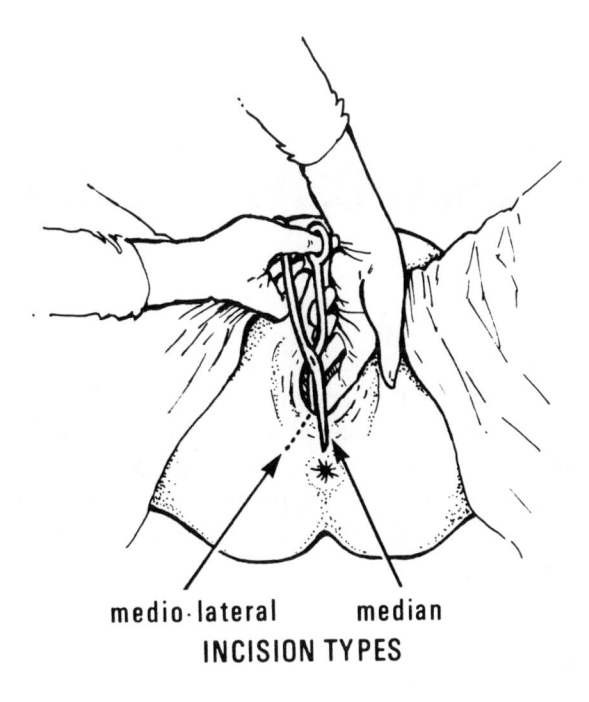

Figure 17.2.   Episiotomy.

Immediate

1. Fetal distress.
2. Delay in second stage of labour.
3. Rigid perineum.
4. To prevent tears in perineal tissue.
5. Forceps or breech delivery.
6. Ante-partum hemorrhage (rare).

Always feel free to discuss this subject with your doctor. Explain that you would prefer not to have an episiotomy if possible. Your doctor will most likely grant your request if there are no complications.

Chapter 18
Cesarean Birth

This chapter will focus on cesarean birth, another way of birthing a baby. Cesarean birth involves the surgical delivery of the baby through the abdominal wall, from the skin to the uterus. The current cesarean birth statistics are high, with a Canadian average of 14.6% to 20%. We shall explore the reasons why the statistics are so high, discuss how one is prepared for cesarean birth, and describe the procedures, the postoperative recovery, and the emotional reactions to birthing this way. In addition, this chapter contains some helpful hints on breastfeeding a cesarean baby, and some postpartum exercises.

WHY A CESAREAN?

Every pregnant woman and her mate should know about cesarean birth, because it can happen to you. Today, the risks of having a baby by cesarean delivery have been minimized due to advanced surgical techniques and anesthesia, the prevention of infection, the use of antibiotics, and the various methods used to control bleeding and manage pain.

Cesarean birth can be an emergency situation, or it can be planned. There are certain situations where you have no choice but to birth this way, as the well-being of both mother and child are taken into account.

MATERNAL HEALTH

Hemorrhaging

Two conditions exist which may cause a woman to bleed profusely while she is pregnant and/or in labour. These are related to the placenta: one condition is called "placenta previa," and the other is called "placenta abruptio." In the first, placenta previa, the placenta has implanted itself over the cervix, or near it. In most pregnancies, the placenta develops from other areas of the uterus, such as the sides, the front or back, or the top. In placenta previa, there is always the risk of hemorrhaging, because if a woman should labour, the presenting part is not the baby, but the placenta. There is no pain associated with placenta previa. The position of the placenta is usually determined by ultrasound, so the cesarean birth can be scheduled; if the woman should labour, it can be an emergency situation.

In placenta abruptio, the placenta detaches itself from the wall of the uterus before the baby is born. This may occur during pregnancy, but it is more often associated with the labour phase. A labouring woman would experience continuous pain in the abdomen, even between contractions. When a health care worker tries to palpate the abdomen, it is very tender to the touch and feels tense due to the pooling of blood. This condition may be concealed if the membranes are intact, or present itself after the baby is born. Excessive bleeding associated with pain is typical of placenta abruptio, and requires an emergency cesarean delivery to control the bleeding. It should also be noted that a placenta may partially detach itself from the wall of the uterus.

Cesarean Birth

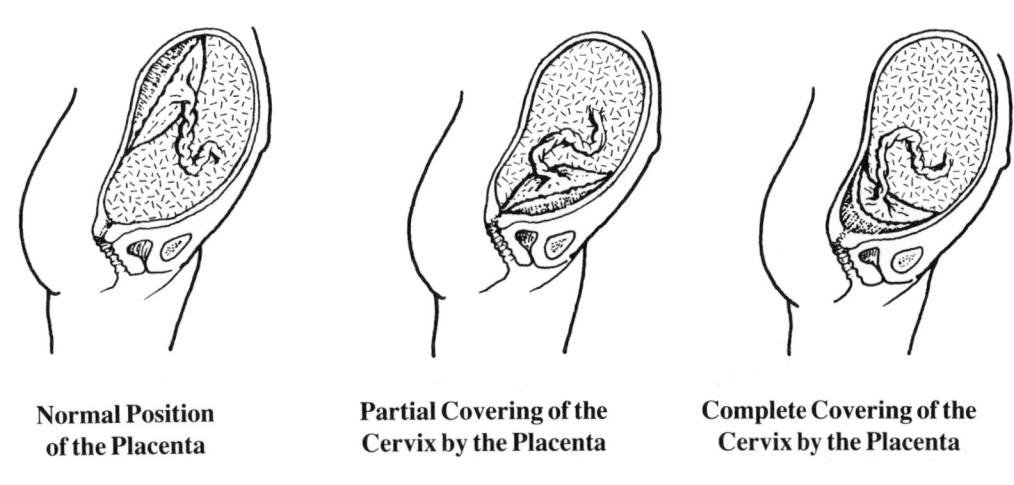

| Normal Position of the Placenta | Partial Covering of the Cervix by the Placenta | Complete Covering of the Cervix by the Placenta |

Figure 18.1. Placenta Previa.

| Normal Position of the Placenta | Detachment of the Placenta from the Uterus (Concealed hemorrhage / Hemorrhage) |

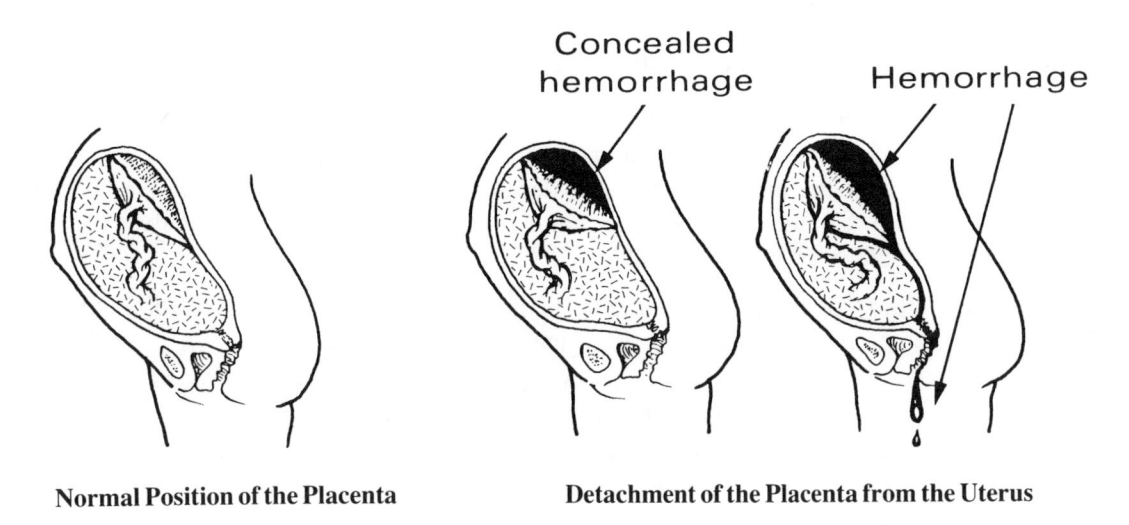

Figure 18.2. Placenta Abruptio.

Genital Lesions

Sometimes, a woman may have lesions in the cervical wall, or in the vaginal wall, preventing her from delivering vaginally. One of these may be cervical cancer. Another condition, such as genital herpes (herpes simplex type 2) may also necessitate cesarean delivery, to prevent the child from acquiring the condition. There are neurological consequences to the child if he should be in touch with the lesions.

Maternal Complications and Risks

Certain women, due to their health, may not be able to deliver vaginally. Cesarean birth is recommended for the safety of mother, the fetus, or both. Women with severe lung or heart disease will deliver by cesarean once the fetus is mature. The diabetic mother may deliver her baby before her estimated date of confinement. Fetal well-being is determined by ultrasonography, non-stress tests, and amniocentesis. Some women with kidney disease may also birth by cesarean.

FETAL HEALTH

Fetal Distress

With the advent of electronic fetal heart monitoring, a fetus who is compromised due to a gradual lack of oxygen can be detected. A small percentage of babies are born by cesarean because of fetal distress. Before the use of the fetal heart monitor, a stethoscope was used to listen to the heart during and in between contractions. This was adequate, but not sufficient to detect the subtle changes in the fetal heart pattern. Changes in the fetal heart pattern will occur, e.g., a decrease in fetal heart rate from the typical 120 to 160 beats per minute to below 100 beats per minute. There is usually a return to the fetal heart baseline. These are usually called heart decelerations. The heart of the fetus may also accelerate, beyond the 160 beats per minute, and then return to its baseline.

Occasionally, the fetal heart rate will descend and stay down at a very low point, such as 60 to 70 beats per minute. The passing of meconium is associated with changes in the fetal heart pattern. A compromised fetus physiologically reacts to a lack of oxygen by passing meconium, his first stools. If the membranes are ruptured, this is easily seen, as the vaginal discharge is green. If the fetal heart pattern is low, and does not return to its usual baseline, then the cesarean birth of that baby is necessary. The reasons for fetal distress may vary; some reasons are given below:

1. Cord Prolapsus: If the fetus is not well engaged in the pelvis, and the membranes rupture, the umbilical cord may slip down into the vagina. The fetus will then press against the umbilical cord and deprive itself of oxygen. A doctor or nurse must push the fetus away from the cord so it can pulsate freely, and deliver the fetus by cesarean as soon as possible.

2. Cord Compression: the umbilical cord may be wrapped once or several times around some part of the fetal body, usually around the neck.

    As a woman labours, the uterine contractions push the fetus deeper into the pelvis, and this stresses the umbilical cord. Fetal distress can result, and cesarean delivery is the solution. Some fetuses are born vaginally with the umbilical cord wrapped around the neck. These fetuses, if they have shown fetal distress, may have been delivered by forceps to accelerate the second stage of labour.

3. Malpresentation: Most fetuses present by vertex, cephalic, or head down (96% of fetuses present this way). Some fetuses present by breech, i.e., buttocks, knees,

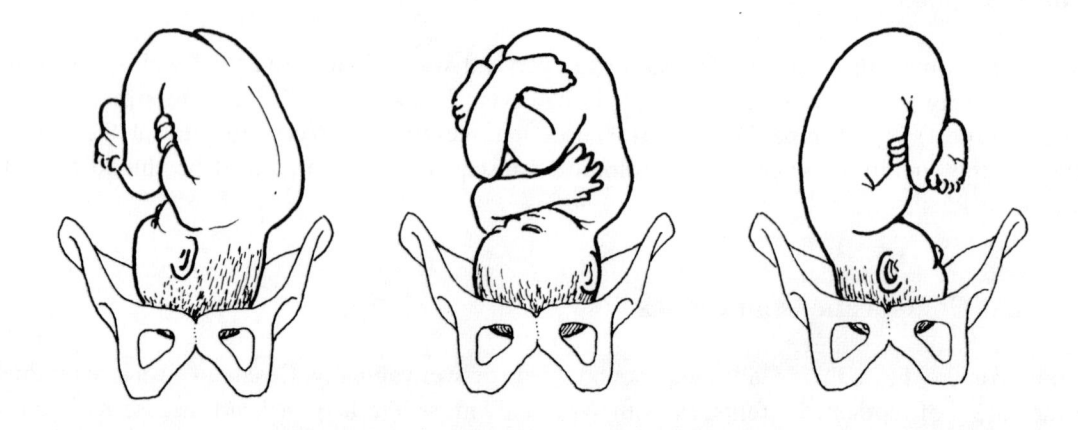

Figure 18.3. Common Presentations (Vertex).

Cesarean Birth 95

Face   **Brow**   **Transverse**

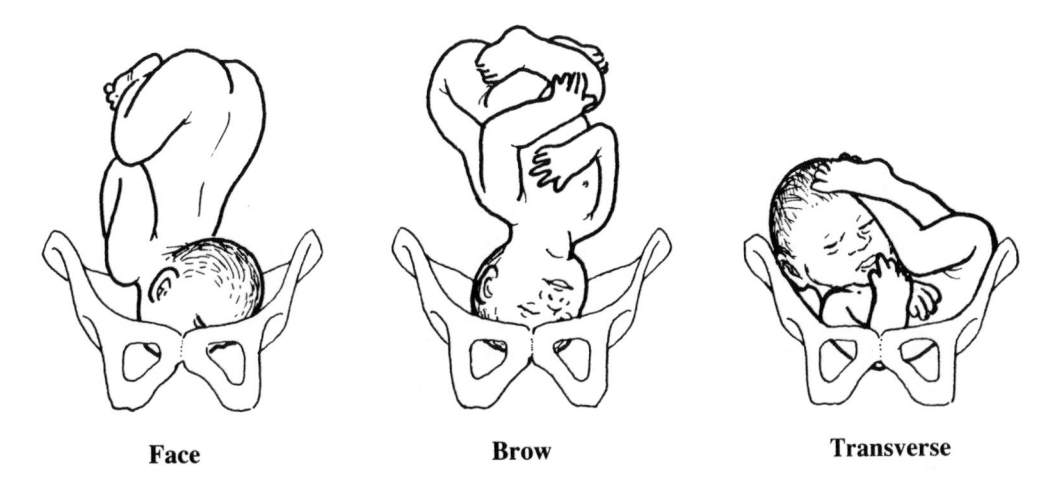

Figure 18.4. Less Common Presentations.

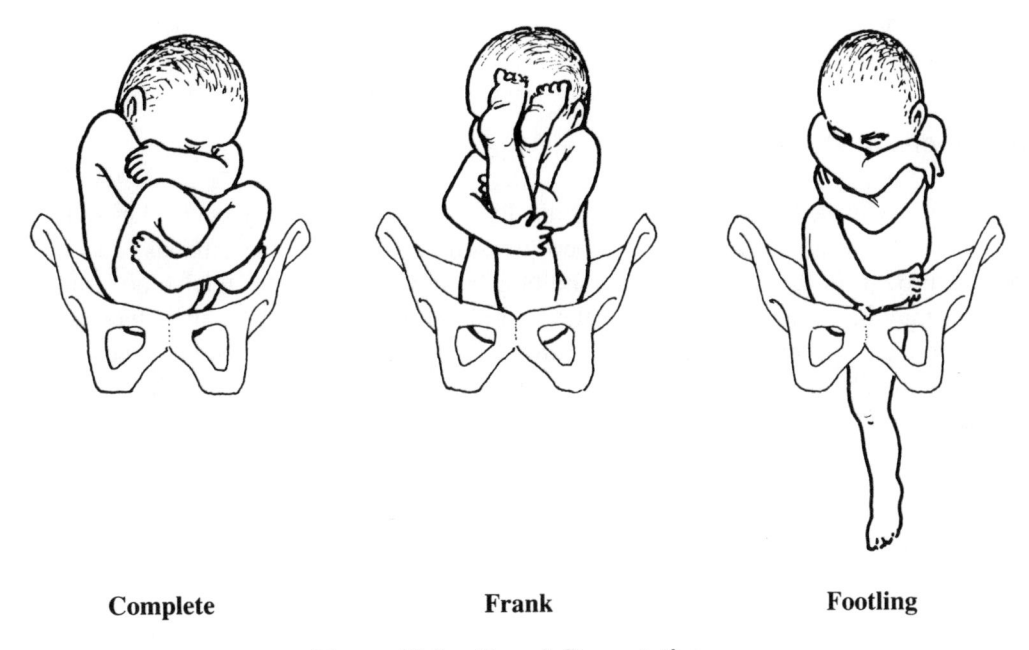

Complete   **Frank**   **Footling**

Figure 18.5. Breech Presentations.

or feet (about 3 to 5% of fetuses are breech presentations). The occasional fetus will present other than in those positions mentioned above; a fetus could be in the transverse presentation (about 1%), or a fetus presents as a combination of parts, such as hands and feet. There are variations of presentations, such as the brow or the face.

If a multiple pregnancy is evident (twins, triplets, etc.), and if one of the fetuses should be a malpresentation, then cesarean delivery is the usual route to follow. Twins which present cephalically will be delivered vaginally.

MATERNAL AND FETAL HEALTH

Cephalo-Pelvic Disproportion (CPD)

CPD is another reason for a cesarean birth. In such instances, a fetus may be too large to descend and pass through the pelvis, or the pelvis may be too small to accommodate the vaginal delivery of the fetus. CPD may be one reason why there is lack of progress, i.e., cervical effacement and dilatation, with labour. The force of the uterine contractions causes the fetus to descend into the pelvis and apply mechanical pressure against the cervix. This pressure against the cervix causes it to efface and dilate. If a fetus cannot enter the pelvis for either of the two above-mentioned reasons, then the cervix fails to dilate, and vaginal delivery is not possible. (See diagram on page 34.)

Uterine Dystocia

Dystocia or abnormal labour accounts for approximately 20% of cesarean births. Dystocia is due to poor uterine function and insufficient contractions which fail to dilate the cervix and move the baby down into the pelvis, or discontinuance of good strong contractions. If certain interventions such as oxytocin stimulation have failed, then cesarean delivery is recommended. Dystocia may also be mechanical, due to CPD.

Complications of Pregnancy

Hypertension or elevated blood pressure (medically called toxemia) may occur during pregnancy or during labour. There is an elevation of blood pressure, swelling of face, hands, and feet, and the presence of protein in the urine. If this condition becomes severe, the fetal blood supply and the oxygenation may be compromised by the elevated blood pressure, with risks of fetal brain damage, and other complications for the mother. Cesarean delivery is one solution. Another condition, prolonged rupture of the membranes for over 24 hours, is associated with increased infection. The mother is at risk for uterine infection, and the baby for septic complications. Cesarean delivery is recommended if vaginal delivery is not imminent.

Previous Uterine Surgery

Some women may be candidates to deliver vaginally, if they had a previous cesarean birth. Other women may need to birth their future babies by cesarean only. Women should consult their doctors to evaluate their obstetrical history, in order to determine if they can be candidates for a VBAC (vaginal birth after a cesarean).

CESAREAN BIRTH ITSELF

A woman must be prepared for cesarean birth when this birthing mode is the choice. Whether the cesarean is planned or an emergency, the steps taken for delivery are the same. The husband or coach is encouraged to be present at all preparatory events as he is able to emotionally support his mate. The following procedures will be performed:

1. Blood Specimens: A health care worker will obtain blood specimens, so that a cross-match of your blood type is available. If hemorrhaging should occur, the

blood bank must have blood available for a transfusion. Also, it is wise to know the level of your red blood cells and your iron content. The anesthetist usually likes to know these results. (N.B. Do you know your blood type?)

2. Intravenous: Because you will be having surgery, an intravenous line is started to provide your body with fluids and as a means of giving you medication, e.g., oxytocin.

3. Consent Forms: When entering the hospital, you have signed a consent form for general treatment. You will now sign for surgery and anesthesia.

4. Shave: to prevent infection, the skin of the abdomen from the pelvic area to the area below the breast is shaved (called a "major" prep). In certain hospitals, only the area below the umbilicus and above the pubic hair is shaved (the "suprapubic" shave).

5. The Obstetrical Team: The obstetrical team is alerted to your cesarean delivery. The team consists of the following:

   - the obstetrician and his assistant, another obstetrician
   - the anesthetist
   - two nurses: one to attend to the obstetricians, and the other to circulate in the operating room
   - the pediatrician
   - mother, father and newborn

6. Preoperative Medication: A preoperative medication is usually given before entering the operating room. All mothers receive one ounce (30cc) of an alkaline-based medication to neutralize the contents of the stomach. This is to prevent damage to the lungs if aspiration of the gastric contents should occur.

7. Vital Signs: Your temperature, blood pressure, heart rate, and respiration rate will be checked at regular intervals.

8. Fetal Heart: The heart rate of your baby will be monitored constantly.

In the Operating Room

Before you enter the operating room, you will wear a bonnet to protect your hair. Once in the operating room, you will be transferred onto the operating room bed. When you enter the operating room, you can expect to see bright lights, equipment for the baby (warmers and resuscitative equipment), equipment for the mother such as monitors and anesthesia equipment, cupboards with supplies, the operating room bed, tables and trays of equipment and linen, chairs and/or stools for sitting, and plastic receptacles. The following procedures will be performed:

1. Cushion: A cushion will be placed under your right side to increase the blood flow to the lower abdomen and prevent compression of the inferior vena cava.

2. Cardiac Leads: Three of these will be placed on you, one on each shoulder, and one near your left breast. These will be connected to a cardiac monitor to verify your heart rate.

3. Blood Pressure Cuff: This will be attached to one of your arms.

4. Position of the Arms: They will be supported by cushions attached to the operating room bed. These will keep your arms perpendicular to your body. If you wish to have your arms or hands free, ask the anesthetist. If you are having regional anesthesia, he may agree. For general anesthesia, it may be necessary to support your arms.

5. Fetal Heart: The fetal heart beat is verified before prepping the skin.

6. Prepping the Skin: The skin of the abdomen from the breasts to the pubic area, the pubic area itself, and the inner thighs will be washed with an antiseptic solution, usually yellowish-brownish in colour.

7. Oxygen Mask: This will be placed on your face till the baby is born.

8. Foley Catheter: Once the skin has been prepped, a foley catheter will be inserted into your bladder, to keep it drained throughout the cesarean, and for 24 hours afterwards. The catheter is attached to a tubing, which is connected to a urine drainage bag. The nurse will keep it drained.

9. Security Belt: A belt will be wrapped around your calves to prevent your legs from rolling off the operating room bed..

10. Draping: Your body and the operating room bed will be draped with sterile linen, to prevent contamination and infection. By this time, the obstetricians, the scrub nurse, and the pediatrician have all scrubbed their hands and arms for five minutes, and have donned sterile gowns and gloves. They will place this sterile linen on you. You can expect to have some of these sheets cover your field of vision, called an "anesthetic drape." This is to prevent you from seeing the surgery. In some instances, the screen may be lowered in order for you to view the birth of your baby. Ask the obstetricians and the anesthetist for this!

11. The Father: While you are being prepared for the cesarean delivery of your child, your husband is also preparing to enter the operating room. Some hospitals encourage the father to attend the cesarean birth of his child in the operating room, so he too must be "prepared." The husband will change from his street clothes into clean linen provided by the hospital personnel. He will then wear paper boots to cover his shoes, a hat to cover his hair, and a mask to cover his nose and mouth. Once the mother has been draped, and before the initial skin incision is made, the father will enter the room, and be guided to sit on a stool at the head of the bed. Here, he also will be protected by the anesthetic screen. You are both free to speak, hold hands, caress each other. The following section will provide the father with information that will be useful to him at the cesarean birth.

The Procedure

The obstetricians will enter by the skin and make an incision here. Two types of skin incisions exist: the "bikini" or Pfannenstiel, and the classical.

The bikini incision is made just above the pubic hair, is slightly curved, and about five inches long. About 99% of the time, this is the type of skin incision that the obstetrician will use. The other 1% of the time, the classical incision is used. Along the midline of the abdomen, from the navel to the pubic area. The other layers will then be exposed, the bladder and nearby tissues identified and separated, and the uterus exposed.

Cesarean Birth 99

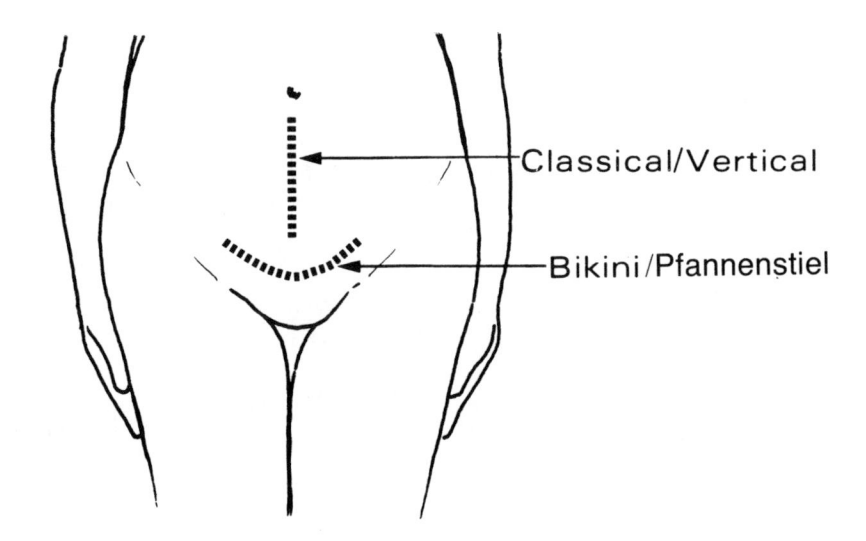

Figure 18.6. Skin Incisions.

- Classical/Vertical
- Bikini/Pfannenstiel

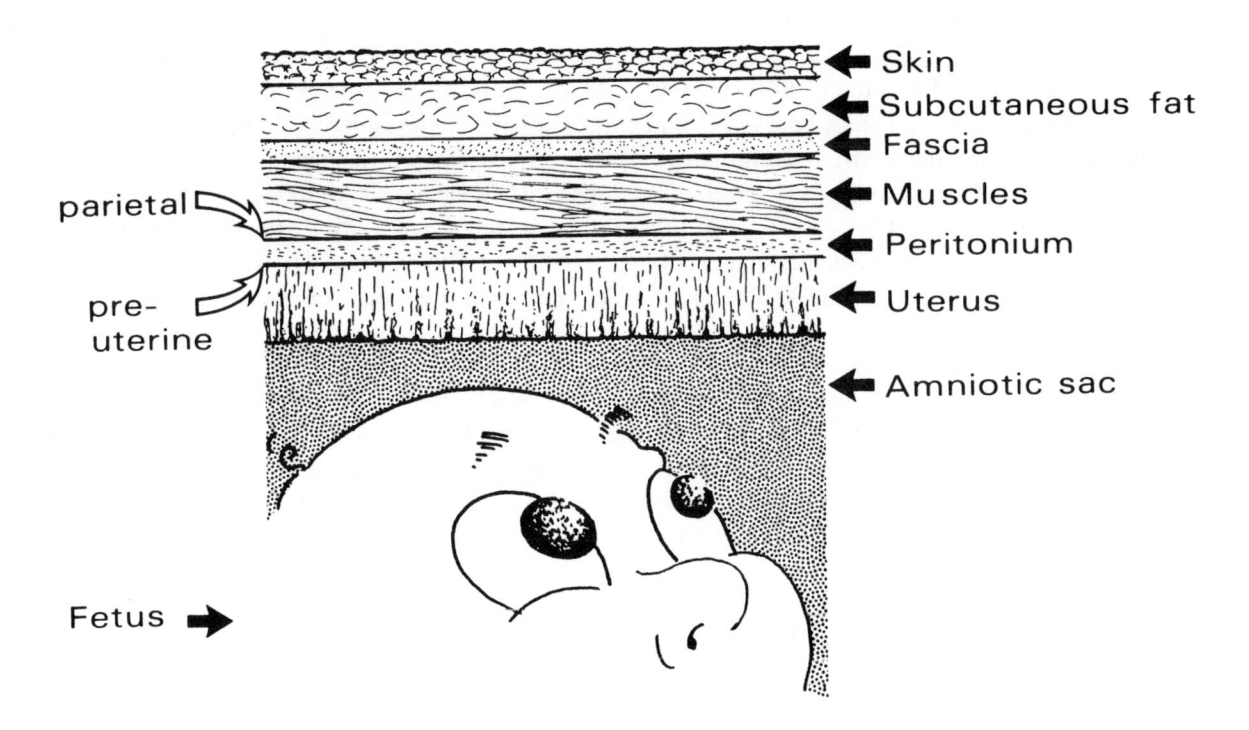

Figure 18.7. The Abdominal Wall.

- Skin
- Subcutaneous fat
- Fascia
- Muscles
- Peritonium (parietal)
- Uterus (pre-uterine)
- Amniotic sac
- Fetus

Two incisions are also possible on the uterus: either a low transverse cervical segmental incision, or the classical. The uterine incision is the low transverse one. In cases of emergency, or if the fetus is premature, a classical or vertical incision is made. It takes approximately five to eight minutes for the abdominal wall to be incised and the uterus opened. The amniotic sac will then be pierced gently,

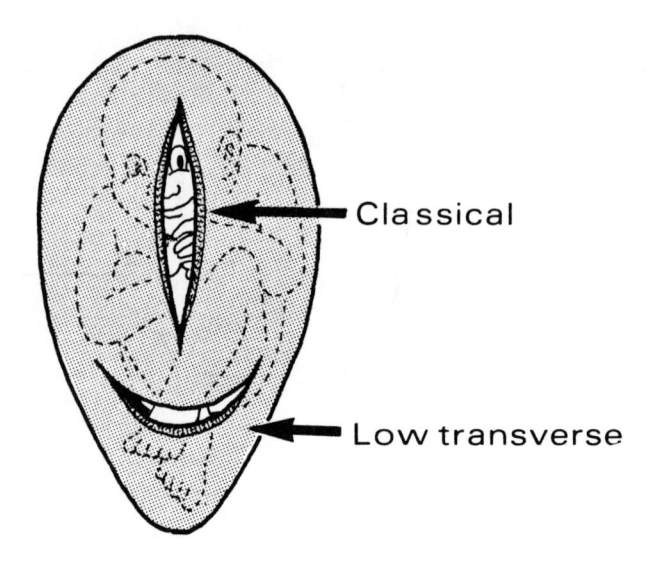

Figure 18.8. Uterine Incisions.

and the amniotic fluid suctioned. The obstetrician will enter the uterus, and using one hand, will lift the presenting part out of the pelvis. He will use the other hand to apply pressure to the top of the uterus (called "fundal pressure") to extract the fetus. Mothers with regional anesthesia often feel gentle tugs and pulls in the birth of the baby. As the fetus is born, the pediatrician will suction the mucus from the oral and nasal passages, and carry the baby to the isolette (a type of incubator). Then he will assess the newborn, suction the baby, and provide oxygen (as needed).

If the baby is healthy, and no complications exist, the baby is wrapped and given to the new parents, to hold, to cuddle, caress, and observe. The obstetricians continue the cesarean delivery, by manually removing the placenta, and cleaning the interior of the uterus. The suturing of all layers of the uterus and the rest of the abdominal wall commences. This may take from twenty minutes to forty-five minutes. The anesthetist continues to monitor the mother's vital signs, and oxytocin is administered to keep the uterus contracting to prevent postpartum bleeding. The skin incision may be closed with a continuous absorbable suture, with Michel clips, or with metal staples. The skin incision is then covered with a dressing. If you are still feeling comfortable and the baby is healthy, you may breastfeed your baby after the birth, either in the operating or in the recovery room. If this is not part of your hospital policy, then you need to ask to breastfeed your baby. Once this is accomplished, you are transferred to the recovery room. Some sounds you may expect to hear in the operating room are:

- The clanging of the metal instruments and bowls
- The suctioning apparatus
- The beeping of the cardiac monitor
- People talking
- Doors opening and closing
- Water running from the faucets
- The intercom system
- Baby's first cries.

ANESTHESIA FOR CESAREAN BIRTH

There are two types of anesthesia: general and regional. General anesthesia is necessary if any of the following are true:

1. There is significant maternal hemorrhaging
2. This is the mother's choice
3. The presence of certain neurological diseases or spine deformities
4. The mother is allergic to certain regional anesthetic agents
5. An abnormal maternal blood clotting process
6. The regional anesthesia is ineffective
7. The anesthetist has not been trained in giving epidural anesthesia.

Regional anesthesia may be necessary for certain mothers with heart and/or respiratory problems. Two advantages of regional anesthesia over general anesthesia is that a mother can be awake and can participate in the cesarean birth of her child with her husband, and that the baby is less prone to respiratory depression. A disadvantage of regional anesthesia is the side effect of hypotension or lowered blood pressure. This can be countered with a generous bolus of intravenous fluids.

General Anesthesia

An intravenous line is initiated, and medication is given to induce sleep (Pentothal), and another (Succinylcholine) to totally relax the muscles of the body. An endrotracheal tube is then placed down the back of the throat so that the mother's breathing can be managed by the anesthetists and to prevent vomitus from getting into the lungs. Once the obstetrician makes the initial skin incision, the mother breathes a mixture of nitrous oxide and oxygen. No more than five minutes are allocated till the baby is born, as nitrous oxide can enter the fetal circulation. For the remainder of the operation, the cesarean mother can receive either a narcotic analgesic (morphine or demerol) or a different gaseous anesthetic such as Enflurane. Once the operation is over, and the mother starts to breathe on her own, the endotracheal tube is removed. Many mothers report that the back of their throat feels sore after the cesarean: this is due to the endotracheal tube if they received general anesthesia.

Regional Anesthesia

There are two types of regional anesthesia: spinal and epidural. In Canada, epidural regional anesthesia is the more favored and practiced by anesthetists, as this form takes more skill and hypotension occurs less often and less severely. Spinal headaches are possible but less frequent (occur in 1% of cases).

The back is washed with an antiseptic solution, and then the skin and surrounding tissue are anesthetized with "local" anesthesia. The anesthetist then feels for the proper entry between the vertebrae, at the lumbar level. With a syringe and needle, the anesthetist applies gentle pressure (this is not painful), till he reaches the epidural space. A plastic catheter is inserted through the needle, and the needle is removed. What remains is a very small plastic catheter, which is held in place with tape and bandages. The epidural catheter is about thirty inches long, and it does trail over the shoulder. It is through this entry (the end near the shoulder) that the medication is given. The typical anesthetics used are of the "caine" family, especially bupivicaine (marcaine) and xylocaine (CO_2). Women report

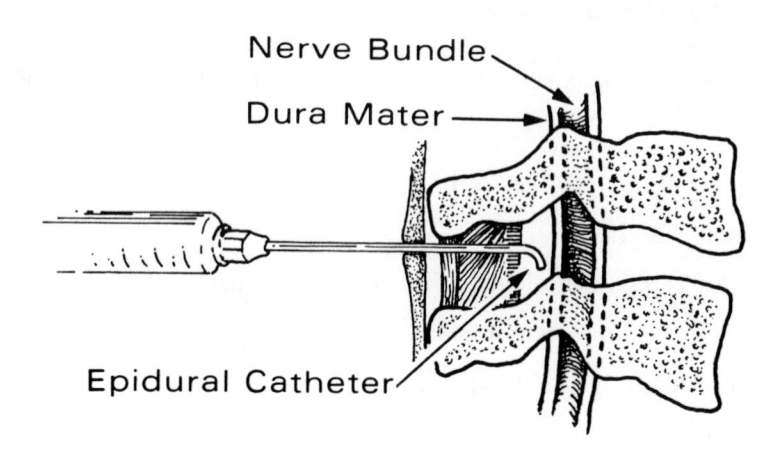

Figure 18.9. Epidural Regional Anesthesia.

feeling warmth in their legs and toes if the anesthetic is effective, and an inability to move their legs. It is normal to experience these sensations. The catheter is removed after the birth.

THE RECOVERY ROOM

You enter the recovery room from the operating room. If you have received general anesthesia, you will be in pain, so pain medication (morphine) is given immediately. You usually feel somewhat sleepy and/or groggy. If you have received regional anesthesia, the effects will start to dissipate one to two hours after its administration. Once you feel sensation return to your legs, especially at the level of the knees, tell the nurse, and she will administer medication for your incisional pain (morphine is used also). The nurse will monitor your vital signs, check the rigidity of your uterus, check the amount and quality of your lochia (vaginal discharge), check your abdominal dressing, and record your intravenous fluid intake and urine output.

You will begin to exercise in the recovery room, to prevent respiratory and circulatory complications. The nurse will first ask you to do deep breathing and coughing, to clear your lungs of their secretions. An alternative to this manoeuvre is saying "ha" several times. Next, you must wiggle your toes, and then rotate your ankles. Once this is done, you will bend your knees, one at a time (with the nurse's support). Try also to lift your arms over your head and prepare your abdominal muscles for mild stretching. One highly recommended exercise is abdominal tightening. This should be done three to four times per hour, every hour while awake. This exercise helps to improve the muscular tone of your abdomen, assists the healing of the incision, and prevents intestinal gas from accumulating. Splint your incision with your hands, inhale, and then, as you exhale, tighten your abdominal muscles. Once you have stabilized and all effects of anesthesia have dissipated, you are transferred to your room on the postpartum unit.

THE FIRST POSTPARTUM DAYS

You can expect the following:

1. The intravenous line is kept in from 12 to 24 hours, depending on your condition.
2. The indwelling catheter which drains your bladder is usually removed within 24 hours.

3. Pain in your shoulders due to blood and air that collect under your diaphragm, and pain due to pressing and irritation of the nerves that go to the shoulders.

4. Pain Medication: If you are breastfeeding, you have to compromise between feeling comfortable and nursing your baby. La Leche League encourages you to take pain medication, as it has little effect on your baby (the effects are not harmful). Take your medication regularly, and if possible, before you expect to nurse your baby. You should also ask for your medication before you arise from your bed, 12 to 24 hours after the birth.

5. Physical Activity: Walk as soon as possible!!! The first time out of bed is the most uncomfortable but the most important. Your instincts will tell you to hunch over, as you try to straighten up from the bed. Your "stiches" won't come apart! Splint your lower abdomen with your hands, as it supports and helps your incision, which feels very tender. At first, you will take short steps, but short steps to a quicker recovery. Also, physical activity *as soon as possible* helps to alleviate problems of intestinal gas common after cesarean delivery.

6. Intestinal Gas: The intestinal tract starts to function within a couple of days of delivery. Simultaneously, you will graduate from sips of water, to a fluid diet, to a soft diet, to a normal diet within three days. Suppositories, an enema, or a rectal tube can help to expel gas trapped in the intestines. Your best solution is physical activity. Certain items should be avoided which trigger or cause further intestinal gas: carbonated drinks (drink only "flat" ginger ale or seven-up, even flat champagne), cold water (drink lukewarm or hot water), certain juices, especially apple, certain foods (like cabbage and broccoli), and caffeine-like compounds (coffee and tea).

7. Lochia: After you have given birth, you will have a menstrual-like flow for a week or two. Try to wear beltless napkins, as the metal claps of the belt may irritate your dressing. Panties which go to the waist are also recommended.

8. Your Incision: The abdominal dressing usually is removed on the third postoperative day, the incision is cleaned and a new dressing is applied. Look at your incision, it can be red and can ooze a little. This is normal. If you have an absorbable skin suture, there is nothing to remove. On the fifth day, half of the clips/staples/silk sutures are removed after the incision has been cleaned. The other half are removed the following day. Sometimes, women report some discomfort with this procedure. If it does occur, ask to be medicated beforehand and/or do some breathing techniques to relax. These should help you.

9. Breastfeeding: Two positions which are helpful for nursing your baby the first two days are (1) the side-to-side position: you are lying down in bed on your side, your back supported with pillows and your baby also lying down on his side facing the breast, and (2) the football position: you are sitting up, and the baby's body hugs your side, and is not across your lap. By the third day, you can nurse your baby quite comfortably sitting up, provided that a pillow is placed across your lap, and another is on the side of your baby. An advantage to breastfeeding for the cesarean mother is the contraction of the uterus via stimulation of the breast nipple—this helps speed the healing of the uterine incision! If you are in bed, and have to change position, place the baby on your chest, and roll together from one side to the other. To burp your baby, simply sit him up, hold his chin, and pat his back.

EMOTIONAL REACTIONS TO CESAREAN BIRTH

For some couples, a cesarean delivery is arrived at after many hours of a long and arduous labour. Many mixed feelings exist for these couples, feelings of joy at the baby's arrival mixed with feelings of frustration and anger. Having a child is complex, both emotionally and physically. A child born by cesarean complicates the situation further. Generally, there are feelings of joy and a relief that the baby has arrived and is in good health. But, if a couple has anticipated a vaginal delivery without "anesthesia," and has assumed the husband would be coaching throughout labour and delivery, the couple feels deprived of something. Some couples have been fortunate to have attended childbirth education classes which prepare them for vaginal and cesarean deliveries, and birth at a hospital which encourages a family-centred approach to cesarean delivery. Feelings that couples experience:

1. Disappointment: This usually occurs with couples who have attended childbirth education classes. They, the couple, have prepared for a special experience, and when their expectations are not fulfilled, there is disappointment. Talk to couples who have had similar experiences.

2. Resentment/Anger: Many women are angry because they laboured for so long and then delivered by cesarean. They often feel less like women because they did not deliver vaginally, like other women. A woman who delivers by cesarean is still a woman. The fact that she is tired and must cope with a new baby after a cesarean, increases her resentment. Men feel angry because they were to participate with their wives in a very long awaited event—the birth of their child. The father usually is not present at the cesarean delivery, so he feels angry towards their hospital and the professional staff. Some couples feel anger towards their babies, because they were the cause of the cesarean. To resolve these feelings, couples need to understand the root of their feelings, and communicate with each other about them. Guidance from a local cesarean support group may be helpful.

3. Fear: Many couples are fearful of cesarean delivery, especially of anesthesia, and the effects of cesarean delivery and of anesthesia on the mother's and baby's health. This quickly passes once the operation is over.

4. Helplessness: Couples who attend childbirth education classes often feel helpless. They have participated in these classes and go into labour with so much enthusiasm. The cesarean delivery takes away all sense of control, so the couple feels helpless. The woman has many things done to her to prepare for a cesarean, and the husband is left outside the operating room, to pace the floor as the fathers did in the "old days." Much of this feeling can be erased by encouraging the couple to participate in the preparation for cesarean delivery, and by having the husband present in the operating room. Feeling *alone* is usually a consequence of feeling helpless. The woman may be the only one in her family or amongst her friends to deliver by cesarean, or the only one in her prenatal group to birth this way. The husband also feels alone because he was not part of the birth event, as other men are currently assisting at vaginal deliveries.

5. Failure: Many women feel they have failed themselves and their husbands by having a cesarean birth. They have such high expectations of labour and delivery, and if these are not met, i.e., by having a cesarean delivery, they have failed. Many men feel they are failures, because they should have participated more as coaches. Feelings of failure can affect the parent-child relationship, because feelings of guilt are mixed in with feelings of failure. Talk with other couples who have delivered

by cesarean. Couples need to establish realistic expectations during the pregnancy, so that the postpartum adjustment is facilitated by a feeling of having coped with the cesarean birth experience.

6. Shock/Surprise: Feelings of shock and surprise typically exist if the cesarean is an emergency, i.e., unplanned, and if the couple has little information on cesarean birth. Some knowledge of cesarean birth, acquired through childbirth education, reading, and speaking with health care professionals, enables a couple to feel prepared for any eventuality.

A note of caution—if many months of consulting with other cesarean couples should be ineffective, and if many negative feelings linger about the cesarean birth experience, seek guidance from your obstetrician or a professional counsellor. A healthy psychological recovery after a cesarean involves an acceptance of the birth experience and the realization that mother and baby are healthy. Feelings of depression can linger for months after the birth. People experiencing such a state of depression need guidance to help them cope with their birth experience.

THE CESAREAN FATHER

The cesarean father is a special person, as he has many demands placed upon him by his wife and new baby. The author conducted a research study, analyzing the impact of cesarean birth on fathers. Twelve men were interviewed on two occasions: the first interview occurring in the hospital, three to four days after the birth of the child, and the second interview three to four weeks after the birth of the child, at home. Two of the subjects were present in the operating room, assisting their wives in the cesarean birth of their children. At the first interviews, the attending cesarean fathers had more positive feelings than the nonattending cesarean subjects about the birth experience and about the health of wife and baby. It was statistically significant that the attending fathers had a greater knowledge base about cesarean birth than the nonattending fathers. In the follow-up interviews, both attending cesarean fathers reported that their attendance at the birth had a positive effect on the subject himself, on his marital relationship, and his relationship with his child. These fathers felt that they had participated in a special event with their wives, and were able to be emotionally supportive to their wives. The support of the obstetrical team at the time of the delivery was seen as important for these two fathers, especially the doctors' explanations of various procedures and encouragement of their participation in the operating room. Both subjects highly recommend fathers to participate in cesarean birth. The fathers are reassured that they need not see the operation, as they are protected by an anesthetic screen. Cesarean childbirth education is encouraged for men who wish to enter the operating room. This is a means of preparing the father for his role in the operating room, and a means to be informed about cesarean birth.

The Role of the Father in the O.R.

The father's role in the operating room is one of physical and emotional support to his wife. During pregnancy, the father should attend the prenatal care visits with his spouse and prepare for his role in the operating room by asking the obstetrician about the possibility of attending the birth. Once in the operating room, the father usually sits on a stool at the head of the operating room bed, near his wife. At this time, he gently takes her hand and strokes it. He should feel free to talk with her and with members of the obstetrical team. Little comfort measures that are appreciated by women are a cool facecloth on the forehead, stroking any part of the head and the arms, talking gently, an occasional kiss, and many words of encouragement. Once the baby is born, an expression of gratitude is appreciated by the woman, a feeling that the couple has shared in something very special. A father's support is needed in guiding the mother through various relaxation and breathing exercises. These encourage the mother to be calm and enjoy the birth event.

Once the skin is sutured, a father is extra helpful when the mother needs assistance for breastfeeding. He is able to hold and guide the child to the breast. Once she is transferred to the recovery room, the father is usually encouraged to follow. Announce the birth to the family and friends! Some hospitals have modified their policies concerning general anesthesia and cesarean birth. Usually in such a situation, the father cannot enter the operating room, but he can receive his child after the birth. The father awaits the child's arrival in the nursery and initiates bonding. A Polaroid camera is useful in recording the baby's arrival to the nursery and provides the mother with an opportunity to envision her child. Fathers can use their humour and imagination in the first few days after the birth. Such a time is difficult for the new mother, and any assistance the father provides quickens the mother's physical and psychological recovery from the birth!

THE RETURN HOME

To assure a healthy physical recovery in the postpartum period at home, the following points are essential to note:

1. Obtaining Help: A woman who must recover physically from a cesarean should only take care of her baby, and leave the housekeeping tasks to another person. It is necessary to obtain help with housekeeping and cooking, at least for the first week. A husband may be helpful with this, but if he is not used to these tasks, the new mother feels obliged to help him. If relatives and/or friends offer help, accept. Any domestic tasks done by them leave the new mother free to cope only with her baby!

2. Physical Activity: A new cesarean mother should avoid climbing stairs for the first week or two. A woman slows her recovery down and easily tires if she must climb stairs, as she is straining the abdominal muscles. There is always concern about lifting weights: the heaviest object that the new cesarean mother should lift is her baby (at least for the first two weeks!). Sometimes, a new mother appreciates occasional medication for pain relief. Before leaving the hospital, she should request a prescription or at least advice from her obstetrician on pain relief. A new cesarean mother should not be left alone with the baby for the first week.

3. Siblings: Young children can feel jealousy once the new mother and baby are home. This is normal. The mother needs to protect her abdominal incision during the first two weeks by avoiding the lifting of young children, and if they should sit on mother's lap, use a cushion as a barrier. Young hands and feet have a tendency to be active and consequently, may hurt mother's lower abdomen. Instructing them to be careful and placing a cushion against the incision are useful in avoiding pain. Engaging siblings in child care and in various activities, such as reading, help them to adjust to the new infant. A very important factor is constantly reassuring the siblings that they are loved and providing physical affection (the "cuddle").

4. Sexual Readjustment: After the first six-week check-up at the obstetrician, the green light is given for the couple to resume their sexual relationship. The man is usually fearful of hurting his partner: the father's participation at this check-up is important to reassure him about this particular point. The vagina doesn't lubricate as well as before pregnancy, so assistance in the form of K-Y Jelly or Lubafax is essential

(intercourse can be very painful if this assistance is not used). These are water-based products, and are helpful in lubricating the vagina. Vaginal secretions are almost non-existent in the lactating female. Certain positions are uncomfortable for the new cesarean mother, especially the missionary or man-on-top position. This usually puts a strain on the abdominal incision. One comfortable position is the side-by-side one. Also hormonal changes can cause a woman to have little interest in sex. Some women report a period of at least four to six months is needed before they feel keen sexual interest. A woman needs much love and foreplay the first few times. Her interest and sexual arousal can be elicited with stroking of her body and other acts of pleasure. Patience and time will lighten these sexual encounters, and the sexual relationship will begin to grow and develop as before the baby's birth. It is not necessary to have sexual intercourse the first time. There are ways to relieve the male of his tension, and arouse the female sexually. Don't rush, but enjoy!

THE BIRTH PLAN AND CESAREAN BIRTH

When preparing for cesarean birth, every couple needs to formulate a birth plan. A birth plan is a constructive tool formalizing the couple's decisions on certain issues, and a means to negotiate with the various members of the childbirth team. Suggestions and recommendations should be sought from other cesarean partners, and from the local cesarean support group. A checklist of options follows, providing the cesarean couple with issues to be discussed:

1. Hospital Admission: Traditionally, when a cesarean is planned and scheduled, the mother enters the day before. Can she enter the same day, and have the cesarean delivery in the afternoon? Can she be permitted to labour and then enter the hospital? Also, for the evening meal, can she and her husband leave the hospital for a couple of hours, and go out to a restaurant for a quiet meal together?

2. Prepping the Skin: Can the nurse perform a partial prep instead of a major prep?

3. Knowledge of Medications: The mother should be aware of the names of medications given, and their effects. Ask for their function.

4. Anesthesia: Seek an interview with the anesthetist to discuss general vs. regional anesthesia. If regional anesthesia is used, ask which type is available in that hospital. Can the mother be awake for the cesarean birth of her child?

5. Father's Presence in the O.R.: Can the father be present in the operating room to witness the birth? Can he stand up and watch the birth of the baby?

6. In the O.R.: Can the foley catheter be inserted after regional anesthesia, when the skin is being washed? Can photographs be taken? Can the mother use a mirror to witness the birth? Can she have her hands and arms free, instead of being tied? Can she have her baby, to see, hold, and touch? Can the father follow the pediatrician to observe the initial care of the baby?

7. Breastfeeding: Can the mother breastfeed the baby in the operating room or in the recovery room?

8. Rooming-in: How soon can a cesarean mother room-in with her baby in your hospital?

9. Recovery Room: Can the father visit the mother in the recovery room? Can he go to the nursery to visit his child?

10. Visiting Hours: What are the hours of visiting for fathers? family? friends? Does the hospital have special sibling visitation times?

11. What is the name of your local cesarean support group?

CONCLUSION

This chapter has presented all the essentials a couple should know about cesarean birth. Cesarean birth is an alternative way of birthing, and with careful planning and proper information, this birth experience can be positive, humane, and warm. Attendance at childbirth education classes that discuss cesarean birth is a first step to being informed. Asking health care professionals about cesarean birth is another way of being informed. Ask, and if you don't understand any specific aspects of cesarean birth, seek counsel and guidance.

Regarding postnatal exercises, you can follow the postnatal exercise program chapter in this book. You can do all the exercises except the one for the abdominal muscles, exercise 4. This exercise should be started six weeks after the birth to allow healing of the incision.

SECTION III:

THE POSTPARTUM PERIOD

Chapter 19
The Postpartum Period

The puerperium refers to the period of six to eight weeks commencing immediately after the placenta (after birth) is expelled. It is completed when the reproductive organs have fully returned to their nonpregnant state. This is a period of rapid recuperation and readjustment after pregnancy, characterized by the following three features:

1. The reproductive organs return to their pregravid (pre-pregnant) state.
2. Lactation (presence of milk in the breasts) is initiated.
3. Recuperation from the physical and emotional experience of childbirth occurs.

The first couple of weeks after the birth of your baby can be very taxing. Just when you are still feeling the exhilaration and probably the exhaustion following the birth of your baby, you may suddenly be overwhelmed by how much is being demanded of you. The care of a baby is no small task, and you may find that you are not as physically strong as you anticipated and that you tire easily. The situation seems to call for the best you can give but physically and emotionally, you may feel exhausted. However, do not despair. This is a time for rest and recuperation and the period during which you will learn the mothering skills.

YOUR STAY IN HOSPITAL

Following the birth of your first baby, you are usually hospitalized for three to four days; and two to three days with your second or subsequent delivery. Following delivery by cesarean, your hospital stay is approximately one week. Of course, this will vary from one unit to the next.

RETURN OF THE UTERUS TO ITS PRE-PREGNANT STATE

Following delivery, the uterus weighs approximately two pounds. However, it quickly shrinks back to its nonpregnant weight of two ounces in about six weeks. Occasionally following delivery, the intravenous solution of dextrose/saline is left in-situ for four to six hours. To this solution may be added oxytocinon —a synthetic hormone which helps the uterus to remain contracted, thus decreasing the likelihood of risk of heavy postpartum bleeding. For the first few days, the uterus feels smooth and hard upon palpation, while its apex lies a few inches below the navel. The marked reduction in its size is most rapid during the first week, at which time it weighs one pound and has descended to two inches above the symphysis pubis (the bone forming the front of the pelvic cavity). By the 12th day after delivery, the uterus is not usually palpable as it has now descended into the pelvis. The process of shrinkage, referred to as involution, progresses more rapidly in mothers who breastfeed. Oxytocinon is released each time the baby sucks at the breast, thus helping to keep the uterus contracted.

VAGINAL DISCHARGE (LOCHIA)

Lochia is the term given to the discharge from the uterus during the puerperium. The amount of lochia varies in different women. It is greater than what is lost during the menstrual flow. There is an odour which is inoffensive. For the first three days this discharge consists mainly of fragments of uterine lining. There may be the occasional small blood clot present. From the 4th to 9th day it is paler and brownish in colour; then from the 9th to 15th day it is yellow-white in colour. Normally all discharge ceases between three to six weeks. Persistent red discharge with foul odour, or the passage of blood clots can be signs of infection. Any such symptoms should be reported to your doctor immediately. While discharge is heavy it is advisable to wear double sanitary napkins. Intra-vaginal tampons such as tampax should not be worn for at least three to four weeks after delivery to allow free drainage of lochia. Of course, these may be comfortable but they can be worn only when lochia becomes less.

INCREASED URINATION

Do not be surprised at the marked increase in urination around the second to fifth postpartum day. During pregnancy your body retains two to three quarts of tissue fluid, and your blood volume is increased. This increased urination is simply a reversal of the process. Some women find it difficult to void because they fear burning and pain, especially if an episiotomy was performed. However, take heart, as after the first voiding all usually goes well. It is important that the bladder be emptied, thus avoiding pressure being exerted on the uterus, which may result in heavy bleeding.

REST AND SLEEP

You may find yourself extremely fatigued after delivery and feel as though you have not slept for days. This is probably true, as you may not have had a really restful night for some time. After you have become acquainted with your baby and are taken to the postpartum floor, the fantastic "high feeling" may begin to wear off. Allow yourself to relax and get a few hours rest, after which you can make those important phone calls. Do not tire yourself unduly with too many visitors. The first day should be restricted to a visit with your husband only. If too many visitors are permitted, you are likely to pay for it with excessive weariness and a depressed "let down" feeling. Make it a point to try to get one to two hours rest during the day, especially after lunch. The importance of getting sufficient rest (at a time when it seems impossible) cannot be overemphasized. Consider your time in the hospital to be a period of rest and recuperation.

Upon discharge, if your baby does not sleep much, try and arrange that someone relieves you while you rest. Share night care of the baby with your husband. Do not feel guilty because he has been working all day; it may not be doing him a favour in the long run. If you become too tired, and you are apt to if you try doing it all, it will affect him too. Do not try to do everything the way you used to. Fatigue may suddenly overtake you, and it may seem as though the whole world is falling apart. Accept assistance from friends who wish to baby sit or help with household chores. If you have a "nursery nurse" or relative helping for the first few days, ensure that you learn the skills of infant care under supervision and don't just be an on-looker. What you really need is someone to help with the housekeeping and to supervise things such as bathing the baby. It's better for you to concentrate upon the direct care of the baby and to leave household matters to the person helping you.

AFTER PAINS

These may begin soon after delivery but rarely last more than two to three days. They are felt as contractions and are usually more severe when the baby sucks at the breast. Such contractions may cause a spurt of lochia or the passage of a small clot. Usually no medication is required but if after pain is severe, mild analgesics can be given at four to six hour intervals during the first two days.

FAMILY CENTRED MATERNITY CARE

Under this system the baby remains at the mother's bedside for the greater part of the time (except when there are visitors other than the spouse). Mother, baby, and father are treated as a unit.

Family centred care is very beneficial for the inexperienced parents. A couple's confidence is built up by carrying out such procedures as changing baby's diapers and bathing and dressing him after these procedures have been demonstrated by the nursing staff. Knowledge gained in this manner is not available when you return home.

Under this system an infant gets more mothering than he would in the nursery. Generally a more satisfactory mother/baby relationship can be established and when dad visits, both parents are more conscious of the family unit. Of course, if you feel tired at any time, the baby can be taken to the nursery while you rest.

AMBULATION

Following delivery you will be kept in bed for four to six hours, thus allowing you some rest. However, it is advisable not to attempt walking alone for the first time after delivery. Following a cesarean birth, you are kept in bed the first day and are helped out by staff on the first post-operative day. Usually, by the third day, you begin feeling more energetic and require little or no assistance in getting around.

LACTATION

During pregnancy the breasts are being prepared for the secretion of milk by the mammary growth stimulating hormones. This is one of the reasons why colostrum can usually be expressed during the ante-natal period. After expulsion of the placenta, the hormone prolactin initiates the production of milk and maintains lactation. However, the true milk does not appear until the second to third day after delivery. When your milk comes in you may feel soreness and discomfort. The breasts now become larger, firmer, hot and sore; the blood vessels in the breasts are more prominent. This is known as breast engorgement. This condition rarely lasts more than 24 to 36 hours. At this time you may feel fatigued and may even have a low-grade fever. However, as the baby sucks, thus emptying the breasts, engorgement subsides. Warm showers as well as a good supporting brassiere are helpful. Mild analgesics also help to relieve the discomfort from engorgement.

In non-nursing mothers, a lactation suppressant medication may be prescribed, depending on your doctor's orders. Some doctors prefer no medications, but it is imperative to support the breasts with a good brassiere. Your doctor may also recommend a restricted fluid intake.

THE CARE OF SPECIAL AREAS

Following delivery you are encouraged to wear double sanitary napkins to absorb the heavy lochia for the first couple days. You are advised to keep the vulva (entrance to the vagina) clean.

Episiotomy

The episiotomy is usually repaired with self-dissolving catgut suture, which means stitches do not have to be removed before discharge from the hospital. Here again, keep area clean and dry. Some doctors prescribe heat lamp treatment to the perineum to improve circulation and help healing of episiotomy. Others prescribe various ointments to be applied to the area, following sitz-bath (soaking of vulva and perineal area in warm clean water). If hemorrhoids have developed during pregnancy, they tend to become rather inflamed and painful after delivery and make a bowel movement a dreaded part of the day. Keep area clean! Heat treatment also tends to be soothing to hemorrhoids, as well as application of anesthetic creams.

Bowel Movement

Ensure that you do not become constipated by drinking plenty of fluids. If necessary, a mild laxative or enema will be ordered. Hands should be thoroughly washed following treatment to perineal area.

Baths and Showers

A warm shower is usually allowed about ten to twelve hours after delivery. If a tub bath is permitted by your doctor, be sure not to add bath salts or fragrant oils, especially if you have had an episiotomy or hemorrhoids, because soapy water entering the uterus can cause infection (the cervix may not be completely closed).

DIET

After the enforced fasting in the labour room, the question most patients ask is: "When do I get something to eat?" If you are hungry and it is meal time, you will be given a general diet of about 3000 calories per day. Otherwise, sandwiches are served with refreshments, or tea and toast. The nursing mother needs a lot of protein and iron and is started on a high protein diet. She is encouraged to drink about four glasses of milk daily. The mother who is not nursing is given a regular diet and is advised to cut down on fluids for the first few days to prevent engorgement.

POSTPARTUM BLUES

It is believed that postpartum blues are caused by rapid changes in hormonal levels and also by the physical and emotional strain of the parenting experience. You may experience it while you are still in the hospital or just after discharge. The new mother often experiences a "let down" feeling. She may become irritable, lose her appetite, and find it difficult to sleep. This may also be related to discomfort (episiotomy, hemorrhoids), baby not feeding well, fatigue, and exhaustion. However, postpartum depression usually passes and is over after a few days. Do not encourage too many visitors, thus tiring yourself unduly. Ensure that you get enough sleep and rest. Upon discharge, confidence must be built up in respect to your ability to care for your baby. Extra help to assist around the house and to babysit while you rest is helpful. This can be provided by a relative or your spouse. Your husband may also experience the blues and will need sympathy. The important issue here is communication. Let your husband know how you feel. Quiz your nurse and doctor and ensure that your questions are all answered. In this way, doubts are smoothed out before you are discharged from the hospital.

EXERCISES

Exercise is important but you should begin moderately. Exercise will restore tone in the over-stretched abdominal and perineal muscles.

RETURN OF MENSTRUATION

The return of true menstruation following delivery will vary in each woman. If you are not breastfeeding, the menses can return between four to eight weeks past delivery. On the other hand, if you are breastfeeding, you may not have a period for eight weeks to one year. However, the average is between four to five months. The amount of bleeding and the interval between periods may be quite irregular for the first five to six months. A woman who has experienced painful menstruation before her pregnancy will often find that the situation has improved.

A point to remember is that breastfeeding should not be included as a form of contraception, since a nursing mother who has not menstruated can still become pregnant if she is not using an effective contraceptive technique.

POSTPARTUM EXAMINATION

Usually, before discharge from the hospital, your doctor will ask you to make an appointment to see him at his office in four to six weeks' time. At this appointment your doctor conducts a full physical examination as well as a pelvic examination, to ensure that the cervix is closed and that there is no infection present. Sometimes, a pap smear is also done as well as a rectal examination to check for the presence of hemorrhoids. This examination gives your doctor the opportunity to ensure that all is well and gives you the chance to ask questions about any problems being encountered. At this time, you can also seek advice concerning the resumption of intercourse, birth control devices, and future pregnancies.

WEIGHT LOSS

The average patient weight loss, one hour following delivery, is about 13 to 14 pounds. Gradually over the first two weeks postpartum, you may lose about 3½ pounds, mainly from the loss of tissue fluid. Even so, you may feel disappointed when you realize you are farther than you expected from your pre-pregnant weight. For this reason try to follow your doctor's advice about not gaining more than the recommended 25 pounds during pregnancy. It can be depressing not being able to fit into your regular clothes, but this can be rectified by watching your diet and eating sensibly. Of course, you are going to be hungry, especially if you are nursing. This is where the conflict comes in, as you are also eager to return to your former shape. Try to stick to your three main meals made up of fresh vegetables and fruits, lots of milk, eggs, cheese, meat, and fish. If you snack between meals, stick to slices of cheese, fruit, yogurt, celery sticks, and carrots. If your weight still bothers you at the end of six weeks, ask your doctor for help. Diet pills are not recommended. These can be dangerous during this time of fatigue and hormonal changes.

THE POSTPARTUM FATHER

The postpartum period is often a time of adjustment for the new father who must deal with the feelings about parenthood at both emotional and practical levels. In addition to his job demands, he now has more responsibility in his home life, and it is therefore quite normal for him to feel insecure in his new role. However, early involvement with baby, as well as love and understanding from you, will make this transitional period much easier for your partner.

The bonding experience between father and baby is just as important as the initial contact between mother and infant. A cuddle from dad initiates that vital first contact and proves that even though the new infant looks very tiny, he is not that frail. Thus, dad's confidence in handling the new baby is given a tremendous boost.

Your partner may be surprised at the amount of time which both of you must devote to the care of the new arrival and he may feel just a little resentful and neglected. The first couple of weeks at home can be just as taxing for dad as they are for you. You are still somewhat exhausted after the birth, but so is he. He has undergone a great deal of emotional stress while awaiting the baby and while assisting you during labour his night's sleep is somewhat interrupted, and he must often wait for his dinner while you tend to the baby's needs.

To ease some of this tension, try to have the baby comfortable when your partner arrives home from work. In this way, you can enjoy time together while you both unwind after the day's activities. If dad does not concern himself with the baby as soon as he walks in the door, this is not a sign of disinterest. He may have had a rough day at work and just needs to relax before playing with Junior.

Allow your partner to become used to the changes gradually and he will soon be taking an active interest in the care of the new baby. He may enjoy activities such as changing diapers and giving Junior his evening bath. While he may appear clumsy at first, try not to be too critical. As time goes on, he will become more proficient at these tasks and, at the same time, will develop a close relationship with his child.

The lines of communication between husband and wife should always be left open so that problems and feelings can be discussed. Issues such as whether or not to breastfeed must be considered. Your partner may not be ecstatic about the idea of sharing this part of you with the baby. Although it may be difficult to discuss some problems, remember that they will not solve themselves. A lot of love and open communication are needed.

You both need time alone with the baby as well as solitary periods. In allowing breathing space with each other, you will come to have a great appreciation for the family unit.

Chapter 20
Postnatal Exercise Program

The following exercises will help you to get back on your feet as soon as possible after the birth of your baby. They are specifically aimed to help you:

1. Maintain good posture.
2. Prevent future back pain.
3. Strengthen your abdominal, pelvic floor, and pectoral muscles.

Begin slowly and do only as much as strength and comfort allow. It is best to start with some of the less strenuous exercises and then work up to the more difficult ones as you become stronger. Repeat exercises 5 times twice daily and work up to 5 to 10 times twice daily.

EXERCISES

1. *Pelvic Tilt:* Lie on your back with knees bent. Tighten stomach, tighten buttocks, and push lower back toward floor. Hold five seconds; relax.

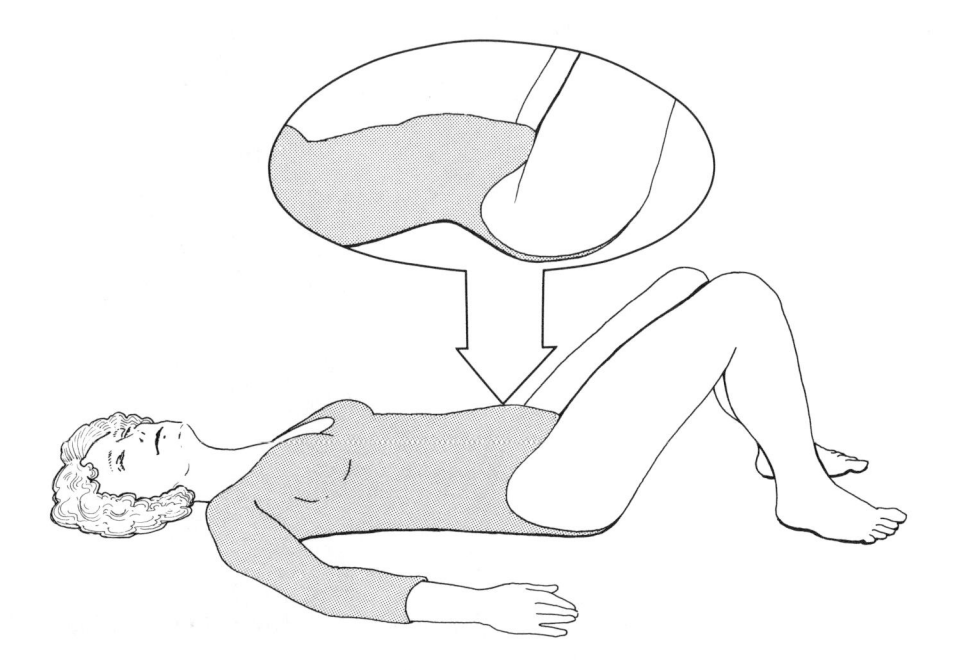

Figure 20.1. Pelvic Tilt.

2. *Leg Sliding:* Lie on your back with a pillow under your head and shoulders. Tilt your pelvis so that the small of your back is pressed down and bend your knees so that your feet are flat on the floor. Slide both legs out until they are straight, then draw them up, one at a time, while maintaining the pelvic tilt.

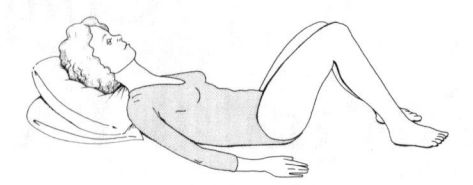

Position 1

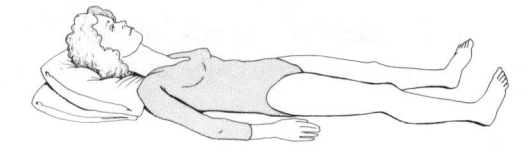

Position 2

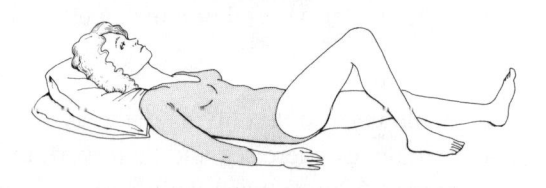

Position 3

Figure 20.2. Leg Sliding.

3. *Pelvic Tilt in Standing Position:* Stand with your back to a wall, feet one step away. Tighten stomach, tighten buttocks, and push lower back toward wall. Hold five seconds; relax.

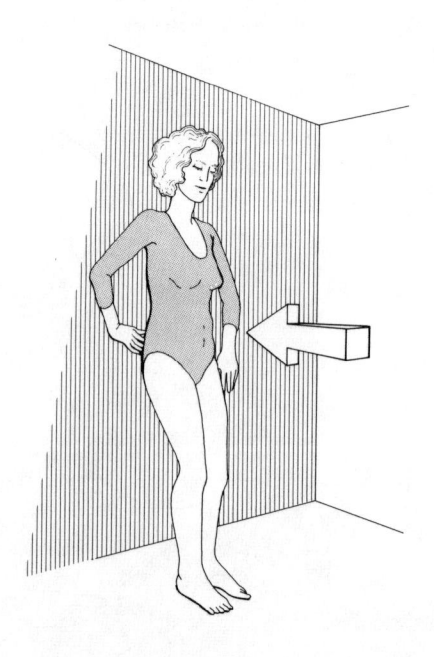

Figure 20.3. Pelvic Tilt in Standing Position.

Postnatal Exercise Program 119

4. *Abdominal Muscles:* Lie on your back with knees bent. Tilt pelvis, tuck chin in, and raise head and shoulders as you:.

   a. stretch hands towards knees, hold five seconds, relax.

   b. stretch hands to the outside of the right knee, hold five seconds, relax.

   c. stretch hands to the outside of the left knee, hold five seconds, relax.

Note: In the event that the rectus abdominus muscle allowed slight protuberance of the abdomen (as mentioned in the Prenatal Physical Exercises, this would feel like a small mid-line bulge when attempting to do an abdominal exercise), you may concentrate on the tilting exercises 1 to 3, above. As the muscle becomes sufficiently stronger, you can begin the abdominal exercises holding your arms tightly around the abdomen.

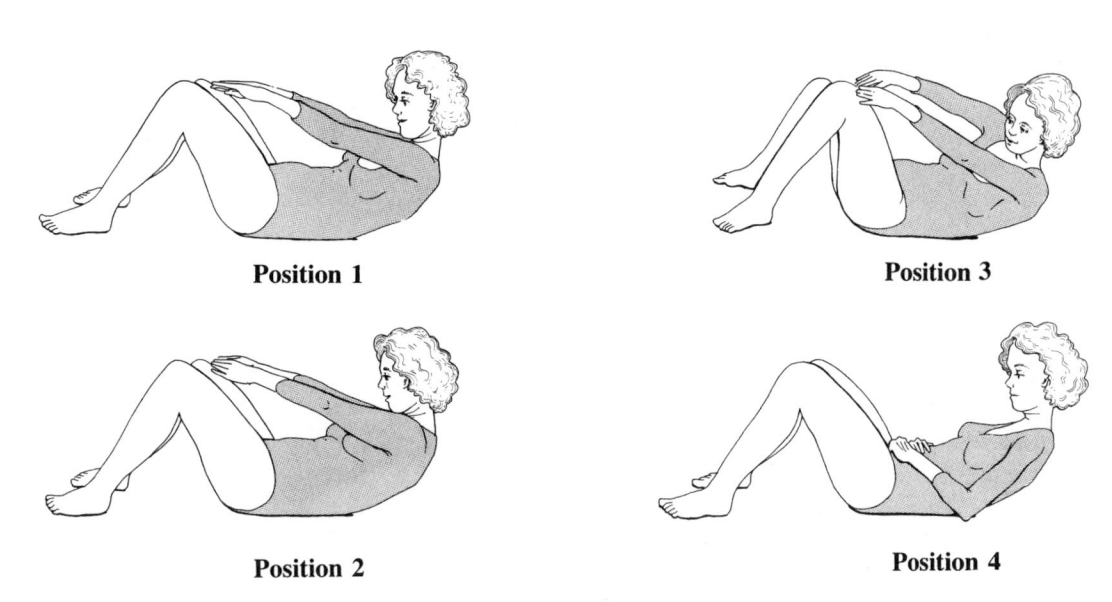

Position 1

Position 2

Position 3

Position 4

Figure 20.4. Abdominal Exercise.

5. *Straight Leg Raising:* Lie on your back with knees bent. Slowly pull one knee up towards chest *(position 1)*, then lift and straighten leg as high as you can *(position 2)*, and slowly bring it down *(position 3)*.

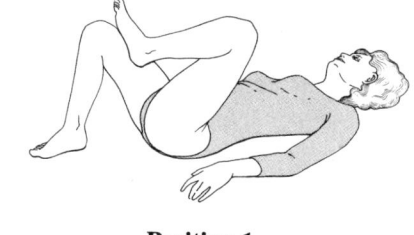

Position 1

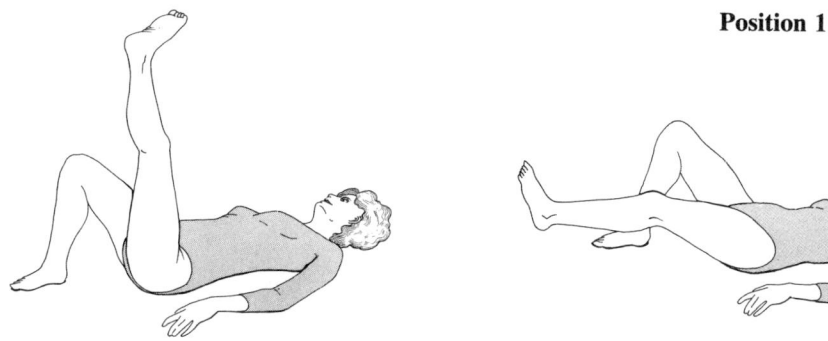

Position 2

Position 3

Figure 20.5. Straight Leg Raising.

6. *Perineal Muscles:*

   a. Lie on your back with knees bent. Tilt pelvis, squeeze knees together, tighten muscles of the pelvic floor, hold two seconds, relax.

   b. Practise stopping urination mid-stream by tightening perineal muscles, hold two seconds, relax.

7. *Pectoral Muscles:* Press hands together in front of your chest, hold five seconds, relax.

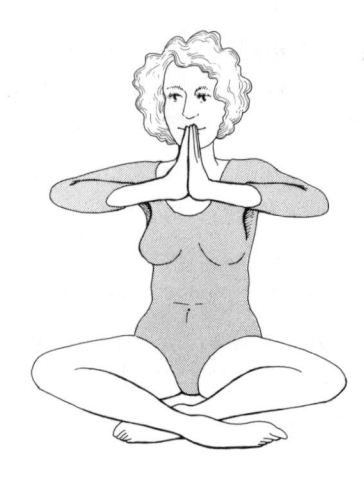

Figure 20.6. Pectoral Exercise.

The above exercises will help you become aware of good posture which should become part of your daily living.

In the first few weeks after the birth of your baby, your back is most vulnerable to stress and it is important to practise these exercises. Of course it is beneficial to continue for the rest of your life. The most important exercises are numbers 1, 2, 3, 4, and 6.

Remember to get enough sleep and rest so you can cope with your new responsibilities.

Cesarean Birth

Mothers who have had a cesarean birth can do all the above exercises except exercise 4. This exercise should be started six weeks after the birth to allow healing of the incision.

Chapter 21
Breastfeeding

The aim of this chapter is to prepare you and your partner for a rewarding experience as the parents of a breastfed baby. As you will discover, the benefits of breastfeeding are numerous. It is also important to note that the father can be an active participant by gaining the information which will enable him to back up and support you in the care and feeding of your baby.

ADVANTAGES TO THE BABY

Since Mother Nature designed the female breast for the purpose of producing milk for the newborn, what better way to ensure your infant receives all the nourishment he requires than the method by which nature intended?

The milk which your body will produce is tailored exactly to the nutritional needs of your baby and is therefore best for him. Nature has created a perfectly balanced supply and demand system which cannot be duplicated. Constipation is almost unknown to the breastfed baby and he is unlikely to get diarrhea.

There are definite indications that breast milk will help your baby to fight off germs that cause disease. It is not known whether antibodies against disease germs are transmitted to the infant through the mother's milk or whether breast milk stimulates antibody production in the baby's system, but the fact remains that breast milk does have certain preventative, protective powers.

No infant is allergic to breast milk, although an allergic reaction may occur as the result of some substance in the mother's food which reaches baby through his milk. When this occurs, the baby is taken off the breast until the offensive food has been eliminated, but he can resume normal breastfeeding after only a few days. It cannot be stressed enough that breast milk is the best food for your baby. In addition, your breastfed baby will gain a sense of well-being, security, warmth, and comfort from the closeness of your body and the skin to skin contact.

A word of caution, however; breastfeeding is beneficial to the baby only if the mother is happy and comfortable about doing so. The mother who breastfeeds only because she thinks it is her duty, communicates her resentment to her child.

ADVANTAGES TO THE MOTHER

As well as the advantages to your baby, there are also many health and fringe benefits of breastfeeding for you. Breastfeeding aids in a more rapid restoration of your figure. As baby sucks on your nipples, he stimulates a certain hormone which will cause your uterus to contract. This helps to expel excess tissue and blood and causes the uterus to shrink more quickly to its pre-pregnant size.

Some cancer researchers believe that a woman who has borne and nursed a child runs a much lower risk of developing breast cancer.

While you are maintaining your infant solely on breast milk, you will rarely ovulate or menstruate. For this reason you are less likely to conceive at this time. However, pregnancies do sometimes occur, so if you wish to plan your family, some form of contraception is recommended.

If it's convenience and economy you are looking for, then breastfeeding is for you. Baby's food is always ready at just the right temperature and it costs you nothing. You will also find travelling less burdensome since you will not have to carry any equipment for breastfeeding.

A breastfed baby also smells nice. His bowel movements and any excess milk that he may spit up are mild and therefore inoffensive to you.

As a nursing mother, you will probably experience a considerable amount of physical pleasure, since suckling a baby gives rise to some of the same physical responses that occur during sexual activity. Thus, you may be more interested in resuming sexual activity than the non-nursing mother. However, in her book *Nursing Your Baby*, Karen Pryor feels that for some women, the opposite is true. Since the menstrual cycle is delayed in nursing mothers, the normal mood swings and peaks of desire are not present. Also, because breastfeeding provides some of the fringe benefits of sex, a woman may turn less often to her husband.

As well as providing physical pleasure, breastfeeding also offers emotional satisfaction and an enormous sense of fulfillment. In the process of nursing your baby, you will form an especially close and interdependent relationship with him. He will depend upon you for sustenance and comfort, while you will look forward to feeding times because of the closeness you will feel towards him, and the pride you will feel in your ability to fulfill his needs in such a loving and intimate way.

THE WORKING MOTHER

If you plan a return to work after the birth of your baby, then you will be pleased to know that it is still possible to breastfeed. Not only is it possible, but also desirable because of the benefits to both of you. While you provide baby with the best possible nourishment, you will both continue to enjoy the special closeness, warmth, and security that only the skin to skin contact of nursing can elicit.

If at all possible, try to remain at home for the first 6 to 8 weeks. This will allow you to form a good nursing relationship with your baby and will ensure the establishment of the let-down reflex and a good milk supply. It is also important at this time that you learn how to express breast milk either manually or with the aid of a breast pump.

After your return to work you can express milk on your coffee breaks and lunch hour to relieve the fullness in your breasts. If you store this milk in a cool place, it can be given to baby the next day. Thus, you will be comfortable and baby will continue to reap the benefits of your milk even when you are not there.

If breast milk is to be stored for more than 24 hours after expression, then freezing is recommended. This is an easy procedure which takes only a little of your time and is a definite convenience. Sterilized containers and covers must be used and milk must first be cooled in the refrigerator before it is placed in the freezer. When adding fresh milk to a partially filled container of frozen milk, it is important to remember to first cool the fresh milk in the refrigerator or freezer to prevent thawing the top layer of the frozen milk. Frozen milk does expand so be sure that the lids are not too tight and the containers are not too full, otherwise they may crack. Frozen milk may be stored for 2 to 3 months and for as long as 6 months under good freezing conditions. To thaw, simply loosen the cap and place the container in warm water. Be sure to shake the container before feeding baby to ensure that the cream is not floating on the top.

As you can see, breastfeeding while working is possible; and you and baby can still enjoy the love, warmth, security, and intimacy which breastfeeding in your non-working hours will afford.

CESAREAN AND PREMATURE BREASTFEEDING

You may be wondering if you can still breastfeed if your baby is born prematurely or by cesarean birth. The response to this question is an emphatic yes. If your baby is premature and is very small, he may have to be fed a high-calorie solution until he is stronger. In the meantime, you can maintain your breast milk by means of manual expression or the use of a breast pump until he is ready to start nursing. If on the other hand, he is just under normal weight and is strong enough to suck, then you may be able to start breastfeeding right away.

Breastfeeding is also possible and desirable for the cesarean mother, as the same hormones which promote milk production after a vaginal birth, are also at work after a cesarean birth. Thus, the milk supply is there, and how soon you begin to nurse depends only upon your condition and the baby's condition following birth. If your doctor and the nurses are aware, in advance, of your decision to breastfeed, they will do everything possible to assist you. If it is not possible to nurse for a day or two, then you can start and maintain your supply of breast milk by means of expression.

BREASTFEEDING TWINS

If you are to be the mother of twins, you may be wondering how you will cope with breastfeeding and whether or not you will be able to produce enough milk to satisfy their nutritional needs. Twins have been successfully nursed by many mothers; and there is no reason why you should not add to this list of happy statistics.

When feeding twins, it is best to alternate each baby on each breast. In this way, even if one twin drinks more than the other, the rate of lactation in both breasts remains fairly even. If however, each twin claims his own breast, there is nothing to worry about except you may be a little lopsided until they are weaned.

You can easily nurse both infants at the same time by holding one on your lap while supporting the other under your arm with the aid of a pillow. You may also want to try tucking a twin under each arm or crisscrossing their bodies on your lap. Or, if you prefer, you may nurse one baby at a time.

JAUNDICE AND BREASTFEEDING

Neonatal jaundice is not uncommon; in fact, 50 to 90 percent of newborns develop some degree of physiologic jaundice. This is normal and need not be cause for concern. The condition is characterized by a yellowish cast in the skin and eyeballs and is the result of the immaturity of the baby's liver function. If your baby has physiologic jaundice, you may continue to breastfeed and the condition will disappear as his liver function matures.

Breastmilk jaundice is a rare condition which appears late in the first or in the second week after birth. Jaundice in the baby is thought to be caused by a substance in his mother's milk. As treatment, some doctors may ask you to stop breastfeeding for 3 or 4 days, in which case you must express your milk until baby is ready to resume nursing. This, too, is not a serious condition and is no cause for concern.

WHY SOME WOMEN DECIDE AGAINST BREASTFEEDING

Up until the early 20th century, almost every healthy mother breastfed her baby. Since that time, a number of cultural changes have altered child rearing trends. Bottle feeding was much more suited to the rigid child rearing practices which emerged at the beginning of the 20th century. At this time, the modern mother, embracing her new liberated identity, did not wish to be tied to the home and children. The baby bottle became a symbol of freedom and the new female identity. Later when the breast was glamorized and viewed as a sexual object, women became embarrassed to breastfeed and many husbands frowned upon the practice because they looked upon their wives' breasts as sex objects to which only they should have access.

Today, however, there is a growing appreciation of the importance of human milk. Young parents are accepting the fact that the breast is best for their baby's psychological and physical needs. In today's modern world, even a working mother can breastfeed. Mothers would be wise to heed the oft-repeated phrase, "It's not the quantity of time you spend with your children, but the quality that counts."

Most healthy women today can, and should, nurse their babies. Breastfeeding is discouraged only if the mother has a serious infectious illness, is taking medication which could be harmful to the baby, or if the infant has some condition which makes it impossible for him to nurse.

Now that you are aware of the facts, and are perhaps convinced that breastfeeding is indeed best for your child, what if, for some reason, you still don't want to nurse him? If the notion of breastfeeding is offensive to you, then don't do it. Your baby would feel your repulsion and resentment and you would be doing more harm than good. Your feelings for your baby are much more important than the manner in which you feed him. An infant who is raised in a loving home is secure and happy regardless of how he is fed.

If you are unsure about your feelings, then why not give breastfeeding a try? You will have lost nothing and can always change your mind if you don't like it. If, on the other hand, you decide to bottle-feed right away, it is much more difficult to change your mind later as it requires a great deal of determination, persistence, and patience.

THE FATHER AND THE NURSING COUPLE

The role of the father is vital to the well-being of the family. For a mother, one of the happiest rewards of nursing is the glow of approval on her husband's face when he sees the baby at her breast.

It takes a little while for a new nursing mother to adjust to her new role. She is vulnerable at this time and needs all the encouragement and support her husband can offer. A mother and father working together to care for their baby is a solid foundation for a close knit, happy family.

ANATOMY AND PHYSIOLOGY OF THE BREAST AND LACTATION

Your breasts are made up of glandular tissue, supporting and connective tissue, as well as protective fatty tissue. The nipple is the pipe line through which your baby will receive his milk. It may be cylindrical or conical in shape and has fifteen to twenty tiny openings through which the milk is secreted. The areola, or dark circle around the nipple, contains the Montgomery's glands, which become enlarged and look like little pimples during pregnancy and lactation. They secrete a substance which lubricates and protects the nipple during nursing. After lactation, these glands recede to their former unobtrusive state.

Let us take a look now at the milk-making structures inside your breasts. The milk is manufactured in grape-like clusters of tiny rounded sacs called alveoli. Each cluster of alveoli is called a lobule, and a cluster of lobules is called a lobe. There are from fifteen to twenty lobes in each breast which are situated at the base of the breast next to the chest. Milk is transported from the alveoli ducts which transport it to the milk reservoirs, located behind the areola.

Breast changes you may expect during pregnancy are as follows:

1. Enlargement and darker colour of the areola.

2. Nipple becomes larger and tender to the touch.

3. Nipples tend to become erect more easily because of stimulation.

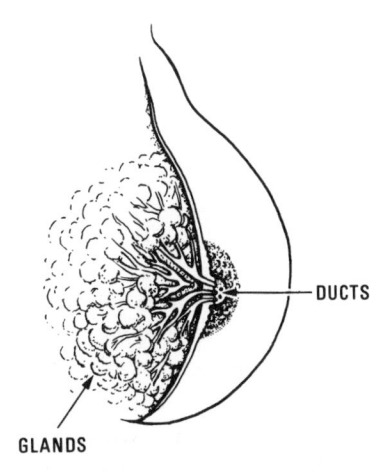

Figure 21.1. Anatomy and Physiology of the Breast and Lactation.

4. Breasts will become fuller and larger until about mid-pregnancy.

5. Milk glands start secreting colostrum (a yellowish liquid) around the fifth or sixth month of pregnancy.

Milk production does not begin until a few days after the birth, but in the meantime, the baby is receiving colostrum, or pre-milk from the breast. Colostrum or pre-milk is what your baby receives before lactation is established. It is an ideal first food for your infant since it is easier for him to digest than true milk. It contains more minerals, protein, vitamin A, and nitrogen, and less fat and sugar. It is also an effective laxative in cleaning out the meconium from your baby's bowels. A changed hormonal balance in your body sets in motion a chain of events necessary for successful lactation. Extra blood is pumped into the small blood vessels of the alveoli causing the breasts to become firmer and fuller. The engorgement and discomfort which this causes in some women is almost always relieved by baby's early and frequent nursing.

Normal milk production is set in motion by your baby's sucking. As he suckles, he is stimulating nerve endings in your nipples, which then send signals to the pituitary gland, directing it to produce the hormone prolactin. Prolactin will keep your ovaries secreting progesterone. For this reason ovulation is repressed and the resumption of the menstrual cycle is delayed. Thus, breastfeeding is a deterrent to pregnancy, but as mentioned earlier in this chapter, it is definitely not a guarantee against it.

As long as your breasts are suckled, they will produce milk. Milk production depends upon a system of supply and demand. If milk is removed from your breasts, they will make more. As the demand is increased, so too is the supply, or production of milk.

The let-down reflex, or milk ejection reflex, is responsible for getting the milk to the baby. Leaking breasts are no longer a problem after the let-down is well established. At this time, the sphincter muscles surrounding the nipple will hold back the milk until your baby begins feeding. When he first sucks, he receives the fore-milk which has collected in the milk reservoirs under the areola. However, it is not until after the let-down that the baby gets the hind-milk containing the fat content which is so necessary for proper nourishment. Human milk differs in appearance from cow's milk in that it is bluish in colour and more watery, but it contains all the nourishment that your baby needs.

As your infant suckles, he is stimulating sensitive nipple nerve endings and is thus setting in motion the process of let-down. The stimulated nipple nerve endings send a signal to the hypothalamus, a tiny structure at the base of the brain, which then instructs the pituitary gland to secrete oxytocin. This hormone then causes the womb to contract.

The let-down reflex may not function reliably during the first days and weeks of nursing. It is a reflex which can easily be hampered by the emotional state of the new mother. Factors such as embarrassment, anxiety, discomfort or uncertainty can, and do, inhibit the let-down reflex.

PHYSICAL PREPARATION OF THE BREAST FOR NURSING

Prenatal nipple preparation is highly recommended as it makes the nipples more supple and conditions them for nursing. Recommended procedures include exposing the nipples to the air and allowing them to rub against outer clothing. This will harden them so that they will not feel as tender when you begin to nurse your baby. Also, try to avoid the use of soap on your nipples as it is drying to the skin. During the latter months of pregnancy, nipple rolling, gentle pulling, and breast massage are recommended. Gentle daily expression (hand milking of the breasts) of a few drops of colostrum is advised as it makes later expression of milk easier and will make you more comfortable in handling your breasts, thus giving you a more positive attitude towards nursing.

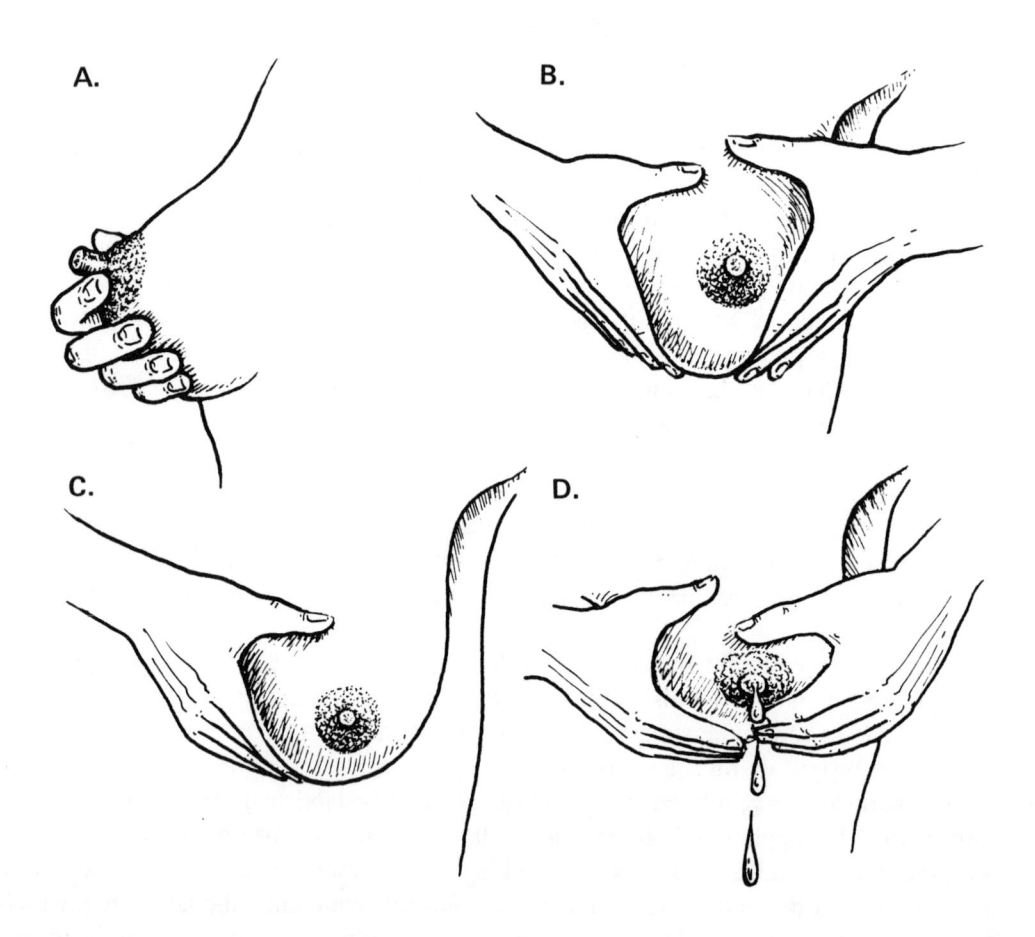

Figure 21.2. Physical Preparation of the Breast.

The technique of manual expression is simple and easy to follow. Grasp your breast just outside the areola with your fingers underneath and your thumb on top. Push down with your thumb against the fingers cupping the back of the breast and slide both thumb and fingers downward toward the base of the nipple, now pull forward and gently at the back of the nipple.

INVERTED NIPPLES

An inverted nipple is one which seems to disappear within the flesh of the breast when the areola is squeezed gently between the thumb and forefinger. Usually, such nipples will protrude by the end of pregnancy and, in almost all cases, will be fully erect when the baby begins to nurse.

The inverted nipple may retract inward with stimulation, thus making it very difficult for the infant to grasp. However, this condition can be corrected by wearing breast cups over the nipple and areola, inside the bra, for increasing periods during the latter months of pregnancy and between feedings after the baby is born. Nursing is still possible even if this condition is not discovered until after the birth. Breast cups have a central opening allowing the nipple to protrude and thus exert gentle pressure and slight suction around the nipple to draw it outward.

SORE NIPPLES

Nipple soreness is common, usually short-lived, and mild, but it can be an unpleasant surprise to a new mother who had not expected discomfort with breastfeeding. Some of the factors which cause sore nipples are: failure to keep the nipples dry, the use of irritating cleansing agents or perfumed ointments, baby's improper grasp of the nipple because of engorgement or other causes, and improperly breaking suction when removing the infant from the breast. Suction may be easily and painlessly broken by inserting a clean finger into the side of the baby's mouth. If these problems continue, soreness can progress to cracking, bleeding, blister formation, and severe pain which will necessitate the temporary interruption of breastfeeding. Management includes a careful search to discover the causal factors and an attempt to alleviate each one.

ENGORGEMENT

The temporary engorgement suffered by some women is caused by the manufacture of milk and vascular expression, which causes the breasts to become firmer, fuller, and very tender. This problem is alleviated by manual or pump expression of milk until the baby is able to grasp the nipple. Frequent and longer feeds also help to empty the breasts. The application of heat before nursing enhances the milk let-down while cold application between feedings will reduce the vascular congestion.

MATERNAL HYGIENE AND BREAST CARE

In order to prevent infection, meticulous washing of the breasts and hands is necessary before each feeding. As stressed earlier, alcohol and soap should not be used on delicate breast tissue since they cause chapping. After feeding cleansing is equally important as it protects the nipple and areola from the growth of harmful bacteria.

To maintain the contours of your breast, it is essential to wear a properly fitted bra. The garment should fit snugly but should not be tight enough to leave marks on your skin and the shoulder straps should be wide and adjustable. You will probably find a nursing bra to be the most convenient since it allows you to uncover one breast at a time without removing your bra. Some nursing bras have plastic liners, which should be removed if they irritate your skin or if your breasts are leaking. The plastic liner will hold in the moisture, thus creating an ideal breeding ground for harmful bacteria which could cause infection.

TIMING OF FEEDINGS

Providing you are awake, the best time to start nursing your baby is as soon as possible or while you are still on the delivery table. Since this will cause your uterus to contract, the delivery of the afterbirth will be accelerated. Also, excessive bleeding will be minimized because the maternal blood vessels which formerly fed the baby are shut off. Research indicates that the infant's suckling reflex is strongest during the first 20 or 30 mintues after birth. If breastfeeding cannot be established in the delivery room, then it should take place as soon as possible thereafter in order that the essential aspects of the sucking reflex and bonding between mother and baby can take place.

Feeding your new infant after he is born for short periods of time is very important to the stimulation of milk production and let-down. Since the breastfeeding infant may be hungry ten or more times a day, it has been suggested that he be placed on a demand schedule or that he nurse every three hours, around the clock.

As breast milk is more easily assimilated into the baby's system than is any other formula, frequent feedings conform more naturally to the emptying of his stomach. The duration of the nursing period is gradually increased by the end of seven to fourteen days, when the final nursing time is fifteen or twenty minutes or more for each breast. Once an infant has become a veteran nurser, he can easily empty a breast within seven minutes, but may enjoy the sucking and the closeness offered by the mother for a longer period.

BURPING THE BABY

All babies swallow air while sucking. The air causes a bubble in the stomach and makes the baby feel too full to take any more milk. Breastfed babies do not swallow as much air as bottle-fed babies, and some breastfed babies hardly ever burp up after a feeding. Others invariably do, often bringing up a little milk in the process.

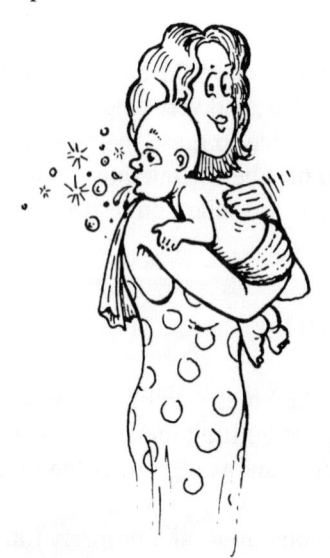

Burping the Baby.

Try burping your baby after he has finished nursing from one breast. If he hasn't burped in a few minutes, don't worry about it. Go ahead and give him the other breast. Try to burp him at the end of the feeding.

To burp the baby, you can hold him upright with his head over your shoulder, and pat his back gently. The slight jogging movement releases the air in his stomach; as the air escapes, the baby burps. Other positions may be used to burp the baby: either sit him on your lap with one hand supporting his head, or lay him on his stomach over your knees. Put a diaper in front of him to catch any spit-up milk.

MATERNAL NUTRITION

There are no specific foods which a nursing mother must or must not eat. A good common sense diet, which includes food from all the food groups, is all that is required to keep both mother and baby healthy. A nursing mother is often very thirsty and should therefore drink as often and as much as she desires. If she does not like milk, she does not have to drink it. However, she should substitute a minimum eight cups per day of other dairy products such as yogurt or cheese.

Baby could be wakeful if mother has had excessive amounts of caffeine, and artificial sweetness may upset his digestion. Sometimes both mother and baby might be affected by a particular food. When this occurs, the mother merely avoids the offensive item and removes baby from the breast temporarily if he has an allergic reaction. A daily vitamin supplement is also recommended.

WEANING

Weaning is the process by which the baby is introduced to other foods and breastfeeding slowly tapers off until he no longer nurses at all. When you give your baby the first supplementary bottle or the first teaspoon of baby food, the weaning process is begun. However, the time at which you stop breastfeeding completely is a decision which must be made by you and your baby. Some mothers nurse for only a few weeks or months while others will continue to breastfeed a toddler. When the decision has been made that you wish to stop breastfeeding, the weaning process should be spread over a period of weeks. In this way, you will suffer little or no discomfort and your baby will have the chance to get used to the idea gradually.

CONCLUSION

While some women may experience mild, temporary discomfort in breastfeeding, the advantages to the whole family make the experience well worthwhile. During the first weeks and months after birth, mother and baby will form a special close bond through skin-to-skin contact, fondling, cuddling, and eye-to-eye contact. The father is also drawn into a closeness, as he is able to support and encourage his wife.

Chapter 22
Bottle Feeding

Infant formula has recently been improved so that it is equal in quality to breastmilk. However, there are many factors, other than nutrition, that aid the physical and psychological growth of a child, such as comfort, stimulation, closeness, and communication. Bottle feeding should be an attitude rather than an action.

ADVANTAGES OF BOTTLE FEEDING

Bottle feeding is often more convenient than breastfeeding, in that it allows the mother more freedom to be away from her baby for longer periods of time.

The bottle feeding mother will be less tired than the breastfeeding mom because her energy will not be drained in nursing around the clock. Indeed, this is one major advantage of bottle feeding, in that dad can share in the pleasure of feeding his child and can easily take over a night or early morning feeding.

It should be added that a combination of breast and bottle feeding is possible once breastfeeding has been well established. If mom wants to breastfeed but has to be away from home part of the time, she may wish to express milk and store it to be used when she is not at home. Formula may also be substituted at this time.

TYPES OF FORMULA

If you choose to bottle feed, using a formula which simulates breastmilk is usually most appropriate. Your pediatrician will recommend a formula such as Similac or Enfalac, depending upon what he feels is best for your baby. If your child reacts adversely to one kind of formula, you may have to change and experiment until you find the one which works for him. Cow's milk is generally not given before the baby is at least six months old.

Table 22.1 summarizes the content of various nutrients in breastmilk, formula, and cow's milk.

EQUIPMENT

Nursers: One set of Playtex, Curity, or Gerber nursers with disposable liners. Disposable liners, while more expensive, are convenient and require no sterilization. The liner collapses as it empties, thus decreasing air intake by the baby. Only sterilization of nipples is required.

Glass Bottles: Eight to twelve 8 oz. bottles and two 4 oz. bottles. Because of the difficulty in sterilizing plastic bottles effectively, glass bottles are recommended.

Nipples: With winged sides. These nipples fill the sides of the baby's mouth to prevent sucking in of air. Nipples should be discarded when rubber becomes flaky.

Bottle Brush

Bottle Warmer

Sterilizer: A large pot or Dutch oven is sufficient. Bottles and nipples should be boiled for 20 minutes, then removed from water immediately to prevent collection of residue. Bottles should be filled as soon as they are cool and stored in refrigerator or freezer. Milk may be frozen for up to six months, and refrigerated for 48 hours.

Bottle Feeding

Table 22.1. Nutritional Comparison

Nutrient	Breastmilk	Formula	Cow's Milk
Protein	Less protein than cow's milk, but easily digestible.	Made easier to digest. Risk of constipation.	Difficult to digest. Risk of dehydration and constipation.
Fats (for energy)	More usable fatty acids.	Depends on type of formula.	Less usable fatty acids.
Cholesterol	High level may help the body to handle this substance later in life.	Lower level than breastmilk.	Low level.
Iron (for formation of red blood cells)	Enough for 2 to 4 months, then a supplement is needed.	Sufficient, if formula is enriched.	Sufficient for 3 months.
Vitamin D (important for growth of bones and teeth)	Sufficient for 2 months if mother drinks enough milk. Supplement needed after this time.	Sufficient if formula is enriched.	Supplement needed after 3 weeks.
Calcium and Phosphorus (important for growth of bones and teeth)	Sufficient.	Sufficient.	Too difficult for kidneys to excrete excess.
Sodium, Potassium, and Chloride (maintain balance in body)	Adapted to needs of baby's immature kidneys.	Similar to breastmilk.	More difficult for kidneys to excrete waste.
Vitamin C (important for structure of tissues)	Supplement required at 2 months.	Sufficient if formula is enriched.	Supplement required at 3 weeks.
Vitamins A and B Complex	Sufficient.	Sufficient.	Sufficient.

N.B.: When feeding the baby, the nipple should always be filled with fluid to prevent air intake. Baby should be burped after every two to three ounces.

INTRODUCTION OF SOLID FOODS

The early introduction of solid foods into the diet of a baby is neither necessary nor beneficial for the following reasons:

- The baby's digestive system is too immature to handle solids effectively until three to four months of age.

- Introducing solids early may predispose to obesity.

- Muscles needed to push food to the back of the mouth do not develop until three to four months.

- Baby needs a lot of fluids. Early solid feeding may reduce his fluid intake.

- The increased fluid intake of protein in the form of meat, plus the decrease in fluids, may harm the underdeveloped kidneys.

- There is more risk of allergy to foods when solids are introduced before three to six months. If either parent is allergy-prone, it is advisable to breastfeed exclusively for six months.

Tips

1. As much as possible, make your own baby food by puréeing cooked vegetables, fruit, and meat in blender or a baby food grinder. This method is cheaper and generally more nutritious.

2. Freeze homemade baby food to save time in preparation. Purée large quantities, then place in ice-trays with individual cubes. Cover, and place in freezer. When frozen, remove from tray and place individual portions in plastic freezer bags.

Table 22.2. Introduction of Solid Foods

Age	Food	Reason
3–6 months	Cereal: first rice, then barley, oatmeal, soy. Start with 1 tsp. of cereal and gradually increase.	Good source of iron, B-vitamins and calories. Commercial baby cereals with fruit added are lower in iron, so are not recommended.
4–6½ months	Vegetables: carrots, beans, sweet potato, peas, squash, broccoli, asparagus, etc.	Good source of minerals, vitamins, flavour and texture. Prevents constipation.
4½–7 months	Meat, fish, poultry, cheese, egg yolk (no earlier than six months).	Source of protein, calories, iron, flavour, texture. No egg white until 1 year—it is more allergenic.
	Fruit and fruit juices (no sugar added).	Source of vitamins, flavour, texture. Prevents constipation.
6–8 months	Texture foods: arrowroot, breadsticks, zweiback, rusks. Peeled apple.	To encourage self-feeding, teething; foods should be lumpier.
1 year	Table food.	Continue to mince meat until child has enough teeth to chew.

3. Do not add cereal to formula in a bottle. Cereal should be served to baby from a spoon. This allows him to practise using muscles of the mouth that he will need to chew harder foods as he grows older.

4. When first giving your child cereal, make the mixture more liquid than solid, then gradually increase the amount of cereal to give a thicker consistency.

5. Do not add sugar or salt to any food or beverage.

6. A vitamin supplement with added fluoride is recommended for babies over two months old.

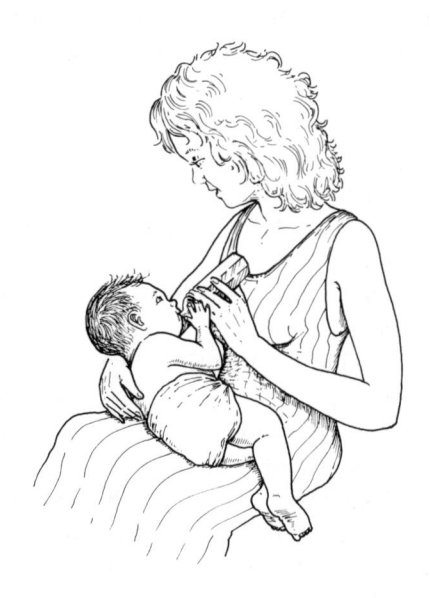

Bottle Feeding

Chapter 23
Infant Care

AT DELIVERY

Several minutes after your child is born, following the cutting of the cord, he will be placed in a warming crib or isolette. There the nurse will wipe off the waxy substance (vernix caseosa) which has served as a protection in his watery environment.

The nurse will examine him briefly, observing his colour, muscle reaction and tone, respirations, and heart beat. She will then bundle him up in a blanket, and give him to you or your partner to hold.

After the placenta has been expelled, and you have had a sponge bath, your new family can spend 20 to 30 minutes together. It is a good time to cuddle and talk to the baby. Studies have shown that a newborn can recognize the voices of both parents. It has also been observed that the child is fully awake for the first hour, and then sleeps deeply over the next 24 hours, so that the bonding process should be initiated as soon as possible.

Recovery rooms are often set aside for this time together, and it is a perfect place to nurse your child for the first time. The nurses are very willing to help you to learn the techniques of breastfeeding, although you need not worry if your infant does not seem interested. After a 12-to-14-hour journey, he can be pretty exhausted, too!

The baby is then taken to the nursery, where he is bathed thoroughly, and dressed in a tiny nightgown. The nurse puts several drops of an antibiotic solution in his eyes to prevent infection.

If you decide to bottle feed, you will probably be given a glucose and water solution for the baby instead of a formula, which will be introduced after six hours.

If you decide to nurse, feel free to ask for your baby as soon as you feel ready and when he seems hungry. The sooner you nurse, the sooner your milk will be secreted. If your child does not seem too hungry the first few times don't panic—he won't starve.

You may keep the child in your room around the clock, if you have a private room. In a semi-private room, the baby can remain with you from the early morning until the last evening feed. However, for their own protection, all babies must go back to the nursery during visiting hours.

In some hospitals, both mothers and fathers can walk into the nursery at any time and pick up their offspring.

You will discover there are classes for feeding, classes for bath demonstrations, and classes for postpartum exercises. These can be beneficial to you, but remember to rest! You will be up from 6 am to 11 pm, with feedings every three to four hours, three meals for yourself, your bath and the baby's bath, and countless phone calls and visitors, sharing in your joy but draining your energy!

Most women having a first child will remain in the hospital three to four days, women having a second will remain two to three days, and women having had a cesarean birth will remain at least five days.

PREMATURE INFANTS

If your child is born prematurely, you may not get the opportunity to nurse him or even hold him in the delivery room. As soon as you are able, however, go to the premature intensive nursery to see him, touch him, and talk to him.

Many preterm infants are not ill babies, but need technological assistance and constant observation to aid them until they reach full gestational age.

You may notice your infant is attached to wires, tubes, and other cumbersome apparatus. Ask the staff what each piece of equipment is used for, and as you spend more time in the nursery, you will feel more relaxed and comfortable in the environment.

You will learn how to hold your child (if he is able to be removed from the incubator) even with the tubes or wires. As you observe and touch your offspring you will discover the slightest of changes, and see them as exciting steps of progress. If you are too tired to come in one day, telephone for an update. The staff are very helpful in giving you information and support and many of them come to love each child they care for.

A baby is usually allowed to go home when he reaches a weight of 2500 gm and is sucking well.

HEAD

You may notice several things about your baby over the first few weeks. Under that soft down you may discover a thick, crust-like substance, usually two to three inches above the forehead. Don't be alarmed! The baby is losing some of his superficial skin layers and as it flakes, it sometimes leaves a residue called "cradle cap." Leave it alone for the first few weeks and if it doesn't go away, take a fine-tooth comb and pass it gently over the cap after a hairwashing. If it persists, try a weak solution of soda bicarbonate. Place one teaspoon of the soda in one cup of water and place on the head overnight. Rinse thoroughly the next morning. Use a minimal amount of shampoo when washing, too, as this sometimes encourages the extension of the cradle cap. If your baby has little or no hair, it may be wiser not to use shampoo at all.

FONTANELLES

You will also discover two soft spots on your baby's skull—one at the back of the head, 2 to 3 cm in diameter, and the other at the front, just below the crown of the head, 4 to 6 cm in diameter. The posterior one will close in 3 to 4 months, and the anterior one in 18 to 20 months. These soft spaces allowed for the overlap of the baby's skull bones during delivery, minimizing pressure on the brain tissue, and allowing for an easier birth for the mother. Many babies are born with heads that have conformed to the shape of the mother's pelvis, and sometimes, in the first few weeks, the baby's head will flatten as it lies against the mattress. It is important to change the baby from side to side after feedings for this reason and because the baby will lose his hair if kept on one side. The fontanelles are covered by a thick membrane so that there is little danger of damage to the brain. It is normal to see the pulse beating beneath the skin in these areas.

EYES

You may be concerned that your newborn's eyes appear unlike anyone's in the family. If the eyelids seem puffy or swollen, it is a result of pressure during delivery and will disappear in two to three days. Are the eyes full of tiny streaks or patches? These are broken blood vessels in the white or schlera of the eye, and also result from pressure. These will disappear within a week or two, if severe.

Why does your baby have blue eyes when everyone in the family has brown? Give him four to six months and he will demonstrate the family traits. Most babies have indigo blue eyes at birth.

The baby may have a slight discharge in the inner corners of the eyes. You can cleanse this with a cotton swab for each eye, dipped in sterile warm water, and brushed from the inner to the outer corners. If the discharge persists or increases, call your doctor. Never use Q-tips.

EARS

These are usually small and well-formed. Cleanse them with a cotton swab or the tip of a facecloth. Again, never use a Q-tip, and never push into the ear. If you notice any discharge, call your doctor.

PHYSIOLOGICAL WEIGHT LOSS

You may notice that your infant is losing weight in the first couple of days. This is not because he is not feeding well, but because he is losing some of the fluids (including blood volume) which he needed in utero, and for labour and delivery. He may lose up to 10% of his birth-weight, but should begin to regain the loss within five to ten days.

PHYSIOLOGICAL JAUNDICE

You may notice a slight yellowish tinge to the baby's skin, two to three days after birth. This tinge may also be apparent in the whites (sclera) of his eyes. Because your child does not need as many red blood cells in his new environment, the body allows the excess to decompose. The end product of this breakdown is bilirubin, but the baby's liver is too immature to filter the bilirubin from the body. With an increase in fluid intake, the child will more readily excrete the waste. If the baby continues to be jaundiced five to seven days after birth, notify your doctor.

MOUTH

You may notice a patchy, white substance on your baby's tongue. This is often caused by milk residue and is referred to as "milk tongue." This may last several days. Do not touch it, as the coating will disappear spontaneously. On the other hand, this may be due to a fungal infection called "thrush." You may notice that the infant has an associated diaper rash. Contact your doctor immediately and he can prescribe a simple medication for treatment.

The baby may develop blisters around his lips after a few days of sucking. These are often seen in breastfed babies, and are caused by pressure due to sucking. They will disappear without treatment and usually will not reappear once the mouth has grown accustomed to the pressure. You may find that your baby has his fingers in his mouth frequently. Putting tiny mitts on his hands will help to decrease the scratching which may accompany this action. Also, it is important to keep his fingernails short, cutting them straight across when the baby is asleep.

BREASTS

The baby's breasts may appear swollen and may secrete a tiny amount of fluid called "witch's milk." This is due to the hormones that the mother has passed on to her child. Do not touch the area, apart from gentle washing, and all will become normal once the child has successfully excreted the hormones.

Infant Care

UMBILICAL CORD

You may wonder what to do with the tiny stump that was once your child's lifeline. Keep it dry and protected. Do not bathe the baby in a tub until the cord falls off in seven to ten days. Fold the diaper beneath the area rather than over it. You can clean it with a cotton swab dipped in a small amount of alcohol or water, but be sure to be gentle while cleansing the base of the cord. Do not use a large amount of alcohol as it will inflame the tissue beneath the base, and dry and flake the skin around the base. Cleansing is only necessary if there is a moderate amount of oozing. You can expect some oozing the first two to three days, but if you notice any bleeding, redness, or a strange odor, call your doctor (it may be infected). Do not pull at the cord—it will detach on its own, and it is not necessary to bandage the area.

PSEUDOMENSTRUATION

You may discover that your tiny daughter has a slightly swollen vulva (the folds around the vaginal opening) and has expressed a few drops of blood. Again, this is because of the hormones she has absorbed from her mother, and she is experiencing a tiny menstrual period! A thick, white discharge may also be excreted and found in the folds of the vulva. Cleanse the area gently from front to back with water only, especially after a bowel movement.

CIRCUMCISION

There are mixed feelings among medical staff whether or not it is beneficial to circumcise male children. Discuss it with your pediatrician before deciding.

After the procedure, the child will have a vaseline-covered gauze strip wound around his penis. This lubricates the tip, and adds sufficient pressure to minimize bleeding. If this drops off, just continue to protect the penis with vaseline only. If there is redness, swelling, or bleeding, call your doctor. A small amount of oozing is to be expected.

You may notice that your son's testicles are not descended into the scrotal sac. This is not unusual in a boy up to one year. Your doctor will regularly check the progress, but mention it to him if you discover they have not descended after that period.

CONSTIPATION AND LOOSE STOOLS

A constipated child will be passing hard, dark stools, infrequently and with great effort. If they are also semi-fluid and semi-transparent, call your pediatrician, as your infant may be underfed.

If your baby is expelling loose stools, is listless, and has no appetite, call your doctor. The child may have an infection.

After each of your infant's bowel movements, cleanse the area thoroughly and pat dry. Corn starch or a lightly perfumed powder is not necessary unless there is a slight redness. A zinc oxide ointment or Ihle's Paste (available at your drugstore) can be applied with a more widespread rash. Often, all that is needed is an "airing" for a few minutes—run the risk of a slightly damp sheet for the purpose of clear skin! If the rash develops into small blisters, notify your doctor.

You may become aware of loose stools when your child is teething. This is quite normal, but extra caution should be taken as the stools are more acidic and can cause a burn to the baby's bottom.

ELIMINATION

Table 23.1. Elimination—Bowel Movements

Type of Stool	Occurrence	Description
Meconium	Initial stool	Black/green, sticky. Necessary for normal digestion to occur.
Transition	2 to 3 days post delivery	Greenish/brown. Combination of meconium and milk stools.
Milk Stool	3 days	Pale brown, formed. More constipation with formula or cow's milk, because of the type of protein, which is less digestible. A small amount of sugar added to formula helps to loosen the stool. Beware of the infant's desire for the sweeter taste. Use sparingly.
Milk Stool (breastfed)	3 days to 3 to 4 weeks	Orangey/yellow liquid paste (sour milk smell) *or* bright green with mucous or curds *or* lemon yellow and watery with curds. The child may take 3 to 4 weeks to reach the accepted orange-yellow, somewhat loose stool. The breastfed baby may have 10 to 12 movements a day, or he may have only 1 to 2 every 3 to 4 days without constipation.
Loose Stool	Teething; ingestion of vegetables or some fruit.	The fruit or vegetable will remain intact. This simply indicates the child is unable to digest the food. Some foods, e.g., grape juice, will colour the stool, causing general alarm. Try to recall food intake before calling doctor.

Elimination—Urination

Your new child may urinate as much as every two hours. Don't be too anxious about changing his diaper every time he goes! A perfect time to change him is before and after a feed. Don't wake him just to change him! Your main concern should be cleanliness and the prevention of diaper rash. Some children are more sensitive to moisture and the chemical properties of urine or your detergent than others. You will learn how sensitive he is after the first few weeks.

The choice of disposable diapers versus cloth diapers usually depends upon the baby's sensitivity. Thorough rinsing of the cloth diapers and not using rubber pants often minimizes rashes.

The baby will urinate less often as he gains more bladder control, and you will realize by five to six months that you are using 12 to 15 diapers daily, as opposed to 15 to 20 at birth. Be sure to clean the perineal area as you change the diaper.

Infant Care

SKIN PECULIARITIES

There are many different spots, colours, and changes you may notice on your baby's skin in the first few weeks.

Do your baby's toes or fingers appear slightly blue? This does not mean, as it would in an adult, that he is not receiving sufficient oxygen, but rather that his circulatory system is immature.

Does your child have little red spots with white centres on his nose, not unlike whiteheads? These milia usually appear within 24 hours after birth, but will disappear in several weeks. This does not mean your child is predisposed to adolescent acne!

The superficial layer of the baby's skin may peel, especially on his hands or the soles of his feet. This is not unlike what takes place after you have had a long, luxurious bath!

Some infants are covered with fuzzy hair, called lanugo. This was necessary as protection in the womb and will shed in a few weeks. It is most noticeable across the shoulders.

HEAT REGULATION

For a full-term baby who is dressed in his diaper and his sleeper with a medium weight blanket, a room that is regulated at 68 to 72 degrees is adequate. A premature baby who has fewer fat deposits may be less capable of maintaining his body heat, and may need more outer clothing or a higher room temperature.

It is not necessary, however, to bundle babies into many layers of clothing. Remember that their body temperature is higher than yours. Observe how you dress and how many blankets you require at night, and outfit your baby similarly. Remember, of course, that he will probably kick off his blankets. A blanket sleeper is ideal for winterwear. If a child appears to get cold at night, warm him up before applying more covers. In covering him while he is still cold, you will lock the colder air in and make it difficult for him to increase his body temperature.

Beware of draughts or wind which might cause a sudden drop in body heat. Be cautious in putting your child in the sun, especially during the summer. Make sure his head is always covered, and that he remains in direct sunlight for short periods of time.

SLEEPING AND CRYING

A newborn may sleep 15 to 16 hours on the average, spending the rest of his time in cuddling, feeding, bathing, or crying.

One of the chief concerns and frustrations of the new parent is dealing with the baby's crying. It can be one of the aspects of parenthood which can lead to tremendous feelings of guilt and failure, if you do not understand the underlying reasons for this action.

Why does a baby cry? Probably one of the most significant reasons is his feeling of insecurity. Everything is new to him. He has left the pleasant warm environment of the uterus and must deal with many new needs and sensations. Smooth, slow motion, cuddling, and rocking often soothe him by providing him with the closeness he needs. A front baby carrier is very effective in calming an agitated baby, combining the movement of the parent and the warmth of the close body. An automatic baby swing (Swingamatic) is often equally effective, although the swing should never be used as a babysitter.

A baby may cry because he may need to fulfill his sucking instinct, in which case a pacifier may suit the occasion. Look for one that is soft for his gums, and one that is malleable to his palate.

Crying is his only way of communicating. Perhaps he is too hot or too cold. Maybe his diapers need changing, or a loud noise or vibration has startled him. Some babies dislike the discomfort of being undressed. Sometimes covering the undressed part with a blanket will suffice.

A cuddle close to the body in a blanket that simulates the closeness and warmth of the uterus might help. Bundle him in a receiving blanket as you may have seen the nurses do in the hospital. Place the blanket like a baseball diamond under the baby, with home base at his head; fold first and third bases over each other, and bring second base up to meet the baby's arms and hands over his abdomen.

Don't pull so tightly that the baby can't breathe, but don't be afraid of a slight tension on the blanket. This simulates his former home, and gives him an immense sense of security.

If he continues to cry, he may have gas pains due to indigestion. If you are nursing, you may have to cut out certain foods which affect your child in this way, such as cabbage, green pepper, onions, chocolate, or spicy foods. By process of elimination you will learn what foods you should avoid. Sometimes, gently pressing the baby's knees to his chest will help to expel gas. If this seems to cause additional discomfort, discontinue the exercise.

If he has fed fairly well in the past one and a half hours, there is a good possibility that he is not hungry, and feeding him again would only increase his distress. However, two to four ounces of boiled water, cooled, might help him feel better.

If you have a child who cries constantly, regardless of initiating the usual comfort measures, he may have colic. This common condition is due to the immaturity of the nervous and digestive systems. The baby may stiffen his body, arch his back, and retract his legs to his chest. He may cry uncontrollably for several hours and any relief may be only temporary. The baby may respond to a warm bath or a gentle massage of the trunk and limbs. You can try to lay the baby lengthwise, with your arm passsing under the chest and abdomen and supporting his head with your hand. The pressure of the arm against his abdomen sometimes alleviates the pain. Gripe water (available at your local drugstore) or a weak peppermint or camomile tea (available at health food stores) can be beneficial. If there seems to be no answer to his upset, position him comfortably in your arms and pace!

Your baby will probably not be sleeping through the night (11 pm–6 am) until he is about three months. If he does so beforehand, be thankful and go to bed at the same time. If he doesn't, wait patiently. Do not follow the advice that two to three tablespoons of cereal at the evening feeding helps to tide him over.

Many babies have a wakeful period each day, often during the evening. This habit may be a difficult adjustment for new parents, who generally consider this the time of the day to sit down and relax. However, it can become an enjoyable time together if you go out for a walk, bathe the baby, or take turns caring for him.

If your baby takes a feeding at 6 pm, and then wakes at midnight to feed and socialize, it may help to wake him at 10 pm instead so that he will be ready to sleep when you are.

A baby will sleep less as he gets older, with his sleep patterns dividing into morning and afternoon naps. Some children sleep two hours in the morning, two in the afternoon, and twelve hours at night. Others manage only one-half hour each naptime. You will become accustomed to your child's patterns, and will be able to discern if he is getting enough sleep. The biggest adjustment comes in organizing your day around your infant's wants and needs. For the first six weeks you may find that there is no particular schedule, but gradually your child will settle into a more established routine.

Remember, your little tyke will not be sensitive to your needs, only to his own! And he cannot express his own needs so you will become an expert at speculation and trial-and-error.

BABY'S REFLEXES AND RESPONSES

You may become startled by your new offspring's twisting, turning, or withdrawals, movements which may appear out of the ordinary.

Let me describe some reflexes which are quite usual. A newborn has a very strong "grasp" reflex, which is probably the most well known of reflexes. This is probably because the new parents can brag about the strength of their child through this response. Dad puts his finger into baby's tiny fist, and immediately the miniature fingers tighten around that large slender object. Dad lifts the child up into the air, on the basis of the baby's strength, and he looks around for the approving exclamations from his friends. Unfortunately, a month later our little guy or gal has lost that Herculean strength! Actually, it is only the reflex that disappears as Junior moves on to other achievements.

If you stroke the infant's hand or foot at the back or the top, the arm or leg will withdraw and the hand or foot will flex and move into a grasping response. This is the "withdrawal" reflex.

The "Moro" reflex is one that results from a sudden change in the environment—a loud noise or bright light. The baby will jump lightly, throw back his head, and arch his back. His arms and legs will flail outward and then return closely to his body, as if to protect himself. He lets out a light cry, and then as if frightened by that cry, will burst into a lusty wail. A whole dramatic episode precipitated by a sudden change!

One reflex can be used to your advantage in feeding your child. If a baby is stroked on one cheek, he will automatically turn toward that side. Often in the first frustrations of feeding, the mother or her helper will grasp the baby's jaw and attempt to direct the baby's mouth toward the nipple. Because of the above natural response, this can be very confusing for the child. Be sure you are ready to insert the nipple into the baby's mouth and then touch him gently on his cheek, and he'll respond with the "rooting" reflex. Touching the inside of the mouth closest to the nipple will also stimulate this response.

Sucking is another very strong reflex and need, something which will start out as a random action as the baby tries to put his fist in his mouth or as he squirms and moves his head in search of an appropriate sucking object. This need decreases as the baby reaches four months.

When placed on his tummy with his face down, he will twist his head to the side to prevent smothering.

Many of the reflexes are a type of protection and are forerunners of activities which will follow with increased maturity. In a sense, the baby is storing these responses in his brain, and they are a learning tool for later development.

Your new baby is not blind. While he may not be able to see distinctly, objects brought within his line of vision (14 to 15 inches) are not a blur. He enjoys colours, and distinctive objects. He begins to focus at about two weeks, and this ability will increase, especially as he sees the same colourful objects which can become imprinted in his memory bank. When we are introduced to a new panoramic view, it is difficult for us to focus on any one thing. How much more difficult it is for a child who has not acquired the skill of organizing and screening his perceptions.

Babies are sensitive to touch and pressure. They will withdraw a foot or a hand if they feel pain. They can sense tension in the person handling them. They feel security in the close comfort of a blanket swaddled about them.

A baby responds to sound. He is startled by loud noises, and yet he can learn to tune them out and may sleep through a barrage of noise in a busy household. An infant prefers rhythmic sounds, music, a soft beating noise, or the hum of an air conditioner.

A baby also enjoys rhythmic movements—that of his mother's rocking body, of a rocking cradle or a baby swing. At his most agitated moments this kind of movement will cause him to be quiet.

When does a baby smile? You will often be told by well-meaning peers or parents that your baby has "gas" or "wind." Actually, it seems that some of those smiles might be practice ones, rather than the force of gas pushing his little mouth open. Some babies have been known to smile quite directly at a specific object at two weeks of age. By four weeks, many are able to distinguish between objects and humans and will respond to the antics of their mother with a smile. Others may not respond until two months. This appears to have little to do with intelligence or contentedness, but is more dependent on how your child is perceiving his environment.

Some babies will begin "talking" sounds at four weeks, while others may "think before they speak"! Remember that your child is an individual who will develop at his own speed, with his own unique personality.

CHOOSING A PEDIATRICIAN

It is essential that you find a pediatrician whom you can trust and who is sympathetic to your feelings about child care. During your pregnancy start searching for a doctor, seeking suggestions from your medical friends, friends who have children, or an obstetrician. It is a good idea, and it is becoming increasingly popular, to make an appointment with the pediatrician before the birth of your baby. It is a good time to discuss your concerns, philosophies, or fears. Having done this, you will feel more secure if a problem arises. If possible, try to find a pediatrician near to your home, although a good doctor is more important than the distance you travel.

You will be given a medical record booklet when you leave the hospital. Your doctor will record pertinent data of your child's progress in this booklet. Your doctor will want to see the baby for his initial visit at two to six weeks of age. Arrange the first visit with the office nurse or receptionist but do not hesitate to call the doctor at *any* time!

BATHING

Initially, handling your baby's slippery body in water may make you nervous, but bath time will soon become a pleasant task for the entire family. Bath time provides a great opportunity for father to spend quality time with his infant. When the baby is a few months old, he and baby may enjoy bathing together in the tub. This close and relaxing time spent with each other will strengthen the bond of caring and love between the two. It will also allow baby to kick and splash to his heart's content, at the same time ensuring his safety in the firm grasp of Dad's arms. This is a fun tradition to establish, and a great prelude to swimming lessons!

You can start bathing the baby as soon as his umbilical cord falls away; until then a simple sponge bath will suffice. Bathing the baby two to three times a week is sufficient, and prevents baby's skin from becoming dry. Less frequent bathing may also protect him from skin rashes. The baby should be bathed at the time of day that is most relaxing and pleasurable for all of you. Bathing baby in the evening before his final feeding often acts to soothe him, so he sleeps longer during the night.

What supplies are needed for the bath? A baby bath is not necessary—your kitchen sink or the bathtub will do the job nicely. A non-perfumed soap is best for your baby's skin. Oils and lotions are generally not recommended unless prescribed by your pediatrician. Have all your supplies close at hand so that you won't have to leave the baby alone during the bath. The temperature of the room and the water should be comfortably warm; avoid draughts, and keep the baby covered when not in the water. Wash the baby from top to toe. One washing of the hair with gentle baby shampoo is sufficient. To wash the hair, the most secure position is to hold him like a football, with his head over the sink, supported by your hand. This prevents water and shampoo from dripping into baby's eyes. When bathing baby, be certain to reach the creases in the neck, the armpits, behind the ears, and the genitalia. It is easiest to lather the baby entirely with soap, using your hand instead of a facecloth, then rinse his skin completely.

Again, don't worry if you feel "all thumbs" at the beginning. Practice makes perfect. Sometimes it's advisable for Mom and Dad to tackle baby's bath time together for the first few months, for moral support.

IMMUNIZATION

Immunization against communicable diseases is essential. Each dosage your child receives should be recorded in his medical record booklet by your pediatrician.

Infant Care

If your child is ill, and is scheduled to receive an immunization, contact your doctor before going to the office. The effect of the vaccine may mask symptoms of the illness. Reaction to the vaccine may take the form of a cold, with fever malaise and a runny nose. You may give your baby Tempra for relief. If you are concerned about any unusual reaction, call your doctor immediately.

Recommended Age	*Vaccine*	*Booster Doses*	
2 months	DPT [diptheria, pertussis (whooping cough), tetanus] Oral Polio	18 months	DPT
		4 to 5 years	DPT
		14 to 16 years	DT
4 months	DPT, Polio		
6 months	DPT, Polio		
12 months	Measles Rubella (German Measles) Mumps		
2 months to 1 year	Tuberculin Test		

LAYETTE

Clothing needs for your baby will vary according to season. A summer baby, for instance, will need more cotton shirts and nighties and less sleepers than a winter baby.

Before investing in clothing and equipment, inquire into borrowing from friends—trading becomes increasingly worthwhile as children grow older. Also, look into second-hand clothing stores and garage sales, where clothing is often nearly new, and very reasonable in price.

Up to one year, clothing should not be of the pullover type. The smallest size you should buy is three months, as sizes are often smaller than the age stated, and your baby will grow quickly.

LAUNDRY

Wash all new clothing before use to remove chemicals which may irritate your baby's skin. Baby's laundry should be done separately from the rest of the family's using hot water and a low perfumed detergent for the wash. Diapers should be soaked in a diaper pail with water and a half cup of vinegar added. For laundering, presoak diapers, put them through the regular wash cycle, then put through the rinse cycle twice.

SAFETY IN THE CAR

It is strongly suggested that a child never be in someone's arms in a vehicle. A baby up to 20 pounds may be strapped in a regulation car seat in the front facing the back. Above that weight, he should be in a car seat, in the back, with the seat attached to a parcel shelf bracket.

He is no longer required to be in a car seat after 2½ years, but must be belted in the back seat until 4 years, at which time he may move to the front.

Check the manufacturer's instructions for placement of seats. In Canada, all car seats are standardized and tested before distribution.

A child should never be in a portable infant carrier or car bed in case of a car accident.

Table 23.2. Layette

Item	How Many	Comments
Sleepers	10 to 12	If you are planning to have more than one baby, good-quality sleepers are much more durable.
Nighties	4 to 6	Sometimes handy in the first few months, as they make the task of changing diapers easier.
Shirts	4 to 6	
Diapers	4 to 6 dozen	Prefolded diapers are more expensive, but are great time-savers.
Plastic Pants	4 to 6 pairs	Best not used continuously, as they may irritate baby's skin. After each change, pants should be rinsed, so that plastic doesn't harden.
Receiving Blankets	3 to 4	Good for bundling baby in the first month.
Sweaters	2 to 3	
Shoes	—	Not necessary until baby starts to walk. Then, shoes with flexible soles, such as good-quality sneakers, are recommended.
Hooded Bath Towel	1	
Crib Sheets	2 to 3	
Blankets	2	
Quilted Changing Pads	2 to 3	
Crib Bumper Pads	1 set	

Some of the above-mentioned items may be changed, according to your baby's needs. You may want to reduce the initial quantity and experiment with how much you need.

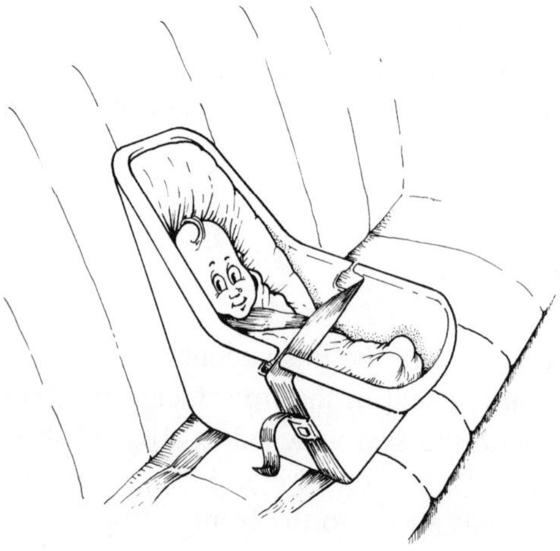

Figure 23.1. Infant Car Seat.

Chapter 24
The Grieving Couple

The subject of grieving is a difficult one to introduce into the maternity setting. Over the past few years, we have learned something of the grief that is experienced by couples whose baby is stillborn or dies shortly after birth. Death at any time is difficult for many to accept but in the labour and delivery room where couples and staff are working with anticipation toward the birth of a baby, it is a very painful experience. The joy, hope, and future are suddenly gone.

At first, there is shock, numbness, denial—"This can't be happening to us." There sometimes is anger, hostility, and blame attached to someone or to the hospital. An overwhelming feeling of guilt settles on some couples. "If only I had stopped working," etc., etc. These are all normal reactions and the couple will need the understanding and support of the professional staff. Occasionally, doctors and nurses have difficulty supplying that support because they also are deeply affected by the death. Even though explanations will be given at the time of death, some may not be understood. At a later date, an appointment should be made with the doctor to talk over any questions that have arisen.

Very soon after the death, couples are asked to make decisions like consenting for an autopsy, whether or not to have a funeral—or see the baby. It seems everything has to be done so quickly and there is no time to make rational decisions. It is true an autopsy should be done as soon as possible to help determine the cause of death but other decisions can usually be delayed. Ask for a few hours to think over these decisions.

There is a great need, after the death of a baby, for the couple to talk over the experience and support one another. Sometimes other members of the family or friends have difficulty expressing their sympathy and concern, perhaps because they have not known or seen the baby. Mothers will say "They never asked about our baby—as if it didn't exist," and will feel angry toward those relatives. Talking about the death seems to facilitate resolution of the grief so relatives and friends can be very helpful by just listening. This baby has to be mourned before the parents can think too much about the future. What is not helpful to hear is "You are young and can have another baby." Mourning takes time—many couples are concerned because they are still mourning months after the death. They dream about the baby and the quality of the dreams can be frightening. They think they are going crazy, and must be reassured that this is a common feeling among couples who have lost babies. In a few months, if things seem to be getting worse—loss of appetite, inability to sleep or cope with household activities—help should be obtained through the doctor. Some hospitals have counselling services which may have been recommended at the time of delivery. Talking with an understanding person is helpful and relieves a lot of the anxiety.

It is important to know the autopsy results, so try to find out who to contact for this information before leaving the hospital. Most final autopsy reports take a few months but a preliminary report is usually available within 72 hours of the death.

Most of the couples we have interviewed after the death of their baby wished they had seen and held the baby. It would seem that the contact helps in the resolution of the grief. Some hospitals take a picture of the baby and this proves helpful when a couple comes and asks if we have anything we could give them that would be a keepsake.

Men and women often mourn differently; women generally mourn over a longer period and a man may not understand why his wife is still talking about the baby. Men have been known to bury themselves in their work but privately cry in the car. Some couples do well just after the birth but have difficulties after a few months. If couples understand that this can be a very stressful period, they will make a greater effort to communicate with one another. Here are two quotations from couples who have lost babies.

> *It was a very special time for me and my husband. We were left with her and we cried together.*

> *The anniversary of his death was very much on both our minds but we hesitated at first to mention it in case the other might not have remembered. . . .*

Most of you who read this book will never have the pain or grief over a lost baby but could, by showing understanding, help others over this life crisis.

Chapter 25
Family Planning

Birth control is now recognized as an essential factor in the protection of family health. The goals of family planning are to help mothers achieve maximum health and well-being between pregnancies, and to rebuild the emotional resources of parents between pregnancies. Child spacing and limitation of family size are now recognized as preventative health measures.

There are many methods of contraception, some relatively new, but most have been in use for centuries. Contraceptive effectiveness depends upon three factors of equal importance: intrinsic value of the method, consistency of use, and proper application. An inferior method used with complete consistency is far better than an effective method used irregularly. Therefore, it is most important that you choose the method most acceptable to you. On these grounds, there is no best method of contraception, but there is a best method for you as an individual couple. The tremendous psychic component in sexual satisfaction makes it wise for you to choose a contraceptive method which you trust completely, which you do not fear because of side effects, and which is not objectionable to you or your partner. Some of the more popular methods of contraception are:

1. Oral pill
2. I.U.D. (intrauterine device)
3. Diaphragm
4. Coitus interruptus (withdrawal method)
5. Condom
6. Rhythm method
7. Non-foaming intravaginal cream, jellies, and tablets
8. Male and female sterilization

THE PILL

The contraceptive pill contains hormone-like substances which prevent ovulation. When used correctly, it gives complete protection from pregnancy. The pill comes in either 21-day or 28-day packages. Described below is the 21-day pill.

1. Day one of your menstrual cycle is the first day you begin to bleed. *The first package of pills must be started on the fifth day* of your menstrual cycle and continued daily for 21 days.
2. Take it at the same time every day when you are most likely to remember.
3. If you forget one pill, take it right away; if possible, the same day. If not, take two pills the next day at the usual time.

4. If you miss more than one pill, use another method of birth control for the remainder of the month, but continue taking your pills.

5. After taking your pills for 21 days, you stop for seven. During these seven days you will probably have a period. If your last pill was on Friday, you start your new package eight days later on Saturday, whether or not you have had a period. Therefore, you will start every new package on the same day.

6. For the first two weeks of the first package, use an additional method of birth control; e.g., foam or condom for added protection.

7. Minor side effects may include:

    a. Nausea

    b. Sore breasts

    c. Spotting (light breakthrough bleeding between periods)

    d. Scantier periods than usual

    e. Weight loss or gain

    f. Changes in your usual vaginal discharge

    g. Depression may occur

If any of the above symptoms persist or you completely miss a period, contact your doctor right away.

THE I.U.D. (INTRAUTERINE DEVICE)

The way the I.U.D. (intrauterine device) works is still not entirely understood. One possibility is that the I.U.D. causes chemical changes in the uterine fluid, adversely affecting spermatozoa, and preventing implantation.

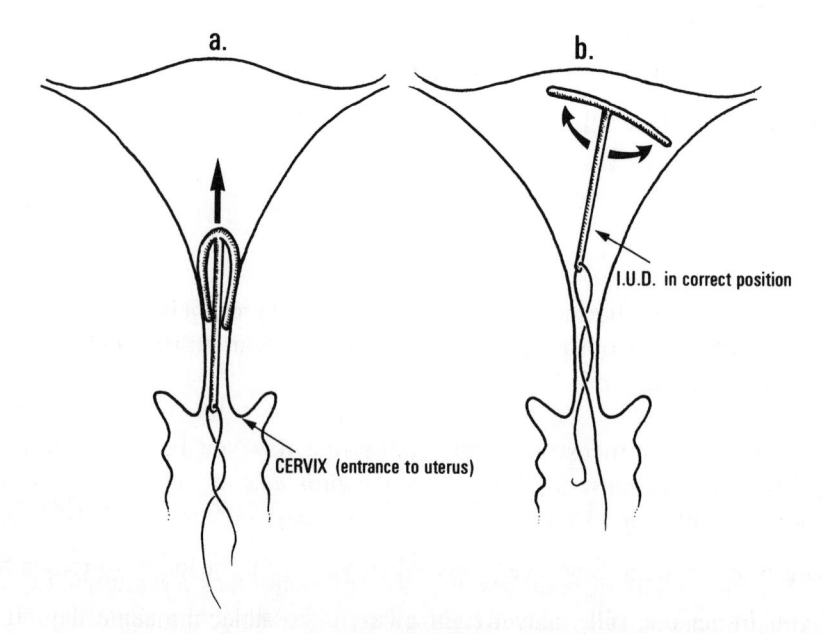

Figure 25.1. Insertion of Intrauterine Device (I.U.D.).

Family Planning

The I.U.D. is a small plastic or metal object that is placed in the uterine cavity. The various types are called loops, coils, rings, springs, and shields. Most intrauterine devices have strings which pass out through the cervix and into the vagina. The presence of the string enables the woman to verify the device is still in place and also provides a means for removing it.

Insertion and Removal

The device is inserted by a doctor, nurse, or technician who places it in the uterine cavity by means of a small tube. It is preferable, but not essential, that insertion be performed during a menstrual period, as the cervix is somewhat softer at that time. The I.U.D. may be used by women who have never been pregnant, as well as those who have. It is usually inserted following pregnancy at your postpartum check-up, by which time the uterus has contracted and the cervix is closed.

Like the pill, the I.U.D. has the great psychological advantage of being disassociated from the act of intercourse. Once the I.U.D. has been inserted, no preparations have to be made or other care taken to prevent pregnancy, thus allowing spontaneity of love making. Usually the string is not felt by either partner. Some notes to remember:

1. Check for the string by inserting the fingers high up into the vagina at least once weekly and after each period. Expulsion may occur even after years of use.

2. For added protection, use foam in addition to the I.U.D. during the fertile period (usually 14 to 16 days before your next menstruation).

3. Minor side effects are:

    a. Cramps and some bleeding after insertion.

    b. Heavier, longer, and more frequent periods for the first few months, as well as backache.

    c. See a doctor for pain, bleeding, fever, or a bad discharge.

If any of the above persist or if the I.U.D. is expelled or should you miss a period, be sure and contact your doctor or clinic. There is a small percentage of patients, about 2% to 3%, who have become pregnant while wearing an I.U.D. Usually this occurs if the I.U.D. has slipped out of place, and for this reason you should check to make sure it is still inserted. Your doctor will also check it at your annual check-up.

THE CONDOM

The condom, often referred to as the rubber, the safe, or the sheath, is a thin membrane which fits snugly over the erect penis. It prevents sperm from entering the vagina during intercourse and provides excellent protection against sexually transmitted infections. Modern condoms very rarely leak or tear. However, it is of utmost importance that the condom be placed on the erect penis before it comes into contact with the vagina. Also, the penis should be removed from the vagina immediately following ejaculation so that the condom does not slip off, thus allowing semen to spill into the vagina.

The condom is a safe device which becomes more effective when used in conjunction with contraceptive foam or jelly. It is relatively inexpensive, may be purchased at any drug store, and is small enough to be carried discreetly. Occasionally, people find it objectionable because they feel it interferes with the spontaneity of their love making or because they are allergic to rubber. In the case of an allergy, the problem is easily solved by switching to a condom made of lamb membrane, called "Skins."

THE DIAPHRAGM

The diaphragm consists of a rubber-covered rim which holds the device in place and of a thin rubber dome which covers the cervix. A spermicidal cream should always be used with it. The dome of the diaphragm prevents the sperm from entering the cervix. The cream destroys the sperm. The diaphragm must be fitted by a doctor after a pelvic examination. Key points concerning the use of the diaphragm:

1. Insert it no longer than two hours before intercourse with jelly on both sides.

2. If four hours pass between insertion and intercourse, inject extra cream into vagina with an applicator.

3. Leave the diaphragm in place for eight hours after last intercourse; remove, wash, and dry well.

4. Do not douche while it is in place.

5. A different size diaphragm may be required after pregnancy or if it is causing discomfort.

6. The diaphragm should be periodically checked for holes and deterioration of rubber. Take your diaphragm with you when you go for your annual check-up.

7. Some women find the diaphragm difficult to insert, inconvenient, or messy. If irritation of the vagina is caused due to the jelly or cream, try changing brands. It is effective and safe if used properly.

COITUS INTERRUPTUS

Coitus interruptus, or withdrawal, is probably the oldest and most common form of contraception. It simply requires that the penis be withdrawn from the vagina before ejaculation. Thus, it is a method which is always available, costs nothing, and requires no preparation or special equipment.

While it is doubtful that the first secretion from the erect penis before ejaculation is responsible for pregnancy, it is known that the greatest concentration of sperm is contained in the first few drops of the ejaculate released at the time of orgasm. Thus, it is the split-second timing required to ensure the effectiveness of this method which also renders it too dangerous.

Coitus interruptus can be psychologically frustrating as the sex act cannot be enjoyed in a relaxed mood by either partner if the uppermost thought is withdrawal in time. This method may also be viewed as inferior because it places total control of both coitus and contraception upon the male partner. However, it is more likely to be successful when there is excellent communication, trust, and respect between partners. Further frustrations may be encountered if orgasm is not achieved as a result of early withdrawal or if postorgasmic closeness is hindered as the result of messy external ejaculation.

RHYTHM OR NATURAL FAMILY PLANNING

The rhythm method requires that intercourse be avoided during the "very fertile" period around the time of ovulation, which occurs 14 days before menstruation. The safe period includes menstruation and the days preceding and following it. It is not harmful to have intercourse during menstruation. The time of the safer period varies, depending on the length of the menstrual cycle. This method is difficult to use if the menstrual cycle is irregular. Women with a regular 28-day cycle can consider

Family Planning

their "very fertile" period to include days 11 to 17, counting from the first day of menstruation. Couples wishing to use this method should maintain records of several factors: basal body temperature, vaginal secretion, and onset of menstrual bleeding. Careful study of these factors will dictate when intercourse should be avoided.

CREAMS AND FOAMS

Creams and foams contain chemicals which destroy the sperm and act as a physical barrier between sperm and the uterus. They should be placed in the vagina by means of an applicator *not more than one-half hour before intercourse*. More of the agent should be injected before each intercourse. Douching should not be performed for eight hours after the last intercourse. Creams and foams are effective if used correctly and consistently, but some find them inconvenient or messy. They may irritate the vagina or the man's penis. Try changing brands if this happens.

MALE AND FEMALE STERILIZATION

Sterilization is by far the most effective means of contraception, but it is also the method which requires the most consideration as it is often not reversible. For this reason, both you and your partner must be absolutely sure that you want no more children, and you must be in complete agreement as to who should have the operation. If either of you have doubts, then it is better to rely upon another method until you are able to clarify your feelings. A hasty decision could well have adverse effects on your relationship and may influence your self-image. That is to say, you may feel like less of a woman or your partner may feel less of a man if procreation is no longer possible. Thus, while sterilization is an agreeable solution for many couples, it is not right for everyone and must, therefore, be given very serious thought.

Vasectomy

Vasectomy, or male sterilization, is a relatively simple operation which is performed using local anesthesia. During this procedure, the vas deferens, or tubes which carry sperm from the testes, are cut and the loose ends are then closed by means of cauterization, a suture, or special metallic tantallum clips. After the operation, the ejaculate appears as before, it is only the sperm cells which have been eliminated.

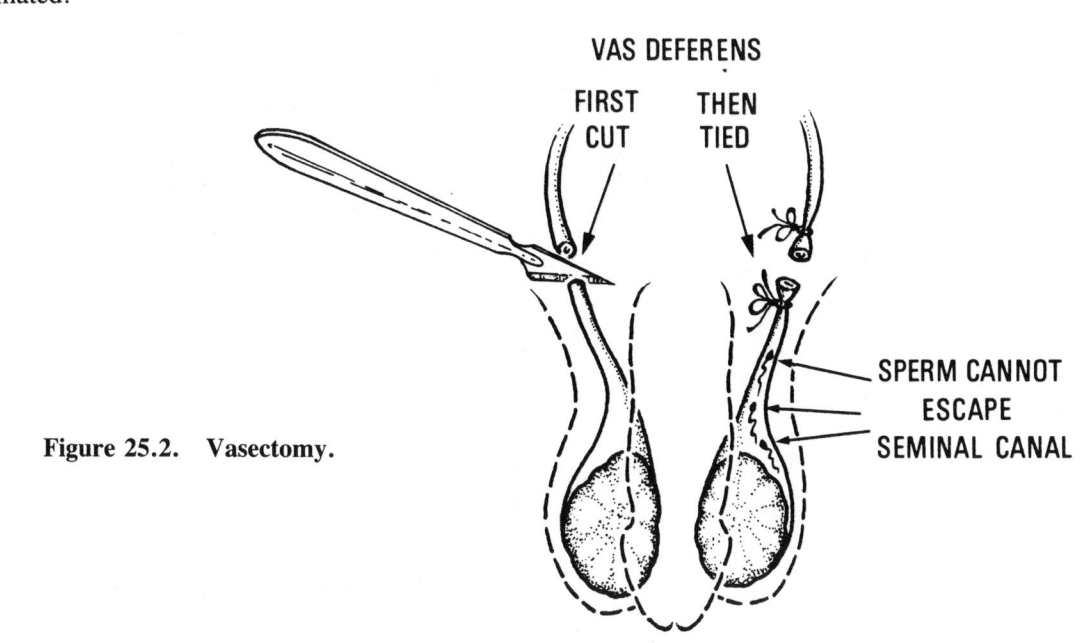

Figure 25.2. Vasectomy.

A vasectomy is usually performed by a urologist in his office, a clinic, or a hospital. You will experience moderate pain on the day of surgery and the day after, and you are advised to wear an athletic support for about a week to protect yourself in the operative area. Depending on the type of job you do, you may return to work within three to seven days and coitus may be resumed within seven days. However, it is of utmost importance to remember that you must continue with your usual means of contraception until the doctor has ascertained that there are no longer active sperm cells in the ejaculate.

In order for the operation to be a psychological, as well as a physical success, a man must be absolutely certain that he wants it. A vasectomy in no way diminishes masculinity, sexual drive, or ability to perform; indeed, the opposite is often true.

Tubal Ligation

Tubal ligation or female sterilization is an operation which involves ligating or tying the fallopian tubes in order to create a barrier thus preventing sperm from fertilizing the egg in the tube. This is accomplished by means of cauterization, the placement of elastic bands and clips around sections of the tubes, or by the use of coagulation. In all instances, a section of each tube must be removed.

Laparoscopic sterilization is the simplest method of performing this operation. The tubes are closed with special instruments through a short incision in the abdomen and only a short hospital stay is required. It may also sometimes be performed on an outpatient basis.

Tubal ligation does not affect the production and secretion of hormones, and menstruation continues as before. The eggs which are released simply disintegrate and are harmlessly absorbed.

As is the case in male sterilization, you should not undergo the operation if you have the least bit of doubt. If you harbour fears of becoming less of a woman or less desirable as a sexual partner, then sterilization is not for you. However, it must be remembered that many women find it to be a happy solution to the problem of contraception. Many report that they feel an increase in sex drive and more desirable to their partners when the fear of unwanted pregnancy has been permanently removed.

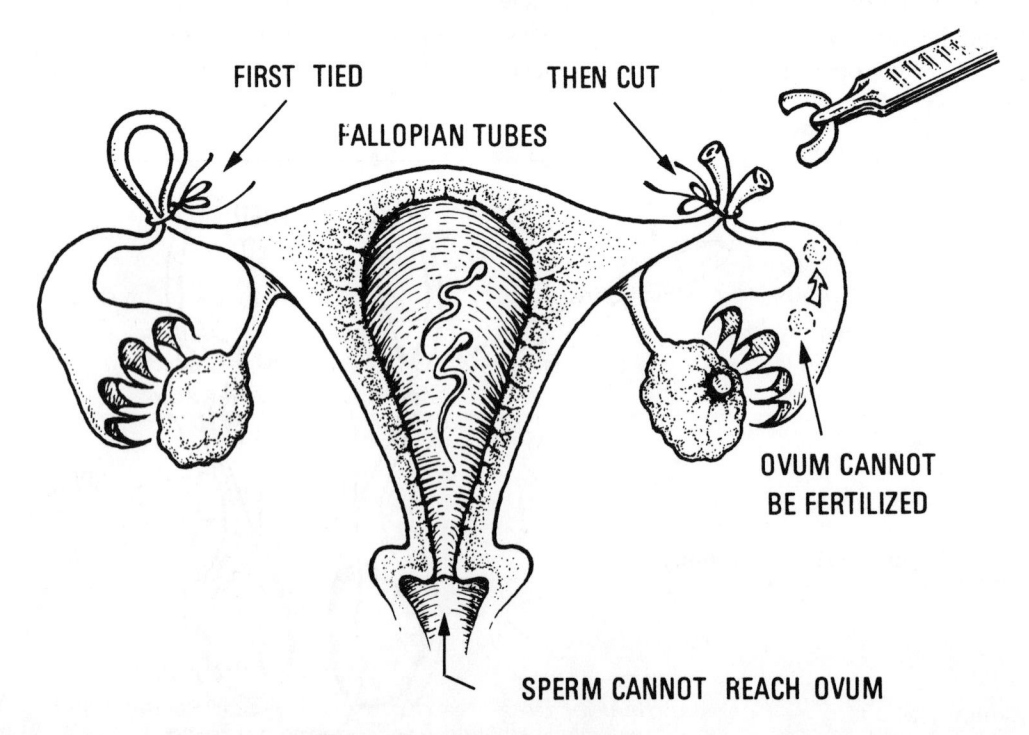

Figure 25.3. Tubal Ligation.

Bibliography

Chapter 3

Canadian Mother and Child—La Mère Canadienne Et Son Enfant. Canadian Health and Welfare.

Comment Nourrir Son Enfant de la Naissance à Six Ans, L. Lambert-Lagacé. Montreal; Les Editions de L'homme.

The Complete Book of Breastfeeding, Dr. Marvin Eiger and Sally W. Olds.

The Family Guide to Better Food and Better Health, R. Deutsch. Creative Home Library, Meredith Corporation.

Feeding Your Child, English Version. Canada Habitex, Collier-MacMillan Canada Ltd. (distributors).

Nursing Your Baby, Karen Pryor.

Pickles and Ice Cream, M. A. Hess and A. Hunt. McGraw Hill.

The Realities of Nutrition, R. Deutsch. Bull Publishing Company.

The Womanly Art of Breastfeeding. La Leche League International.

Chapter 4

Flanagan, Geraldine. *The First Nine Months of Life.*

Kitzinger, Sheila. *The Complete Book of Pregnancy and Childbirth.*

Montague, Ashley. *Life Before Birth.*

Nillson, Ashley. *A Child is Born.*

Verny, Thomas. *The Secret Life of the Unborn Child.*

Chapter 5

Bourne, Gordon. *Pregnancy*, Pan Books, London and Sydney, 1978.

Greenberg, M., and Monis, N. "Engrossment: The Newborn's Impact Upon the Father," *AMJ Orthopsychiatry* 44: 520-531, 1974.

Hines, J. "Father, the Forgotten Man," *Nursing Forum* 10: 177-200, 1971.

Kitzinger, Sheila. *Education and Counseling for Childbirth Educators*, Schocken Books, New York, 1979.

Mitscherlich, Alexander. *Society Without the Father*, Schocken Books, New York, 1970.

Chapter 6

Bing, Elizabeth and Colman, Libby. *Making Love During Pregnancy.*

Hotchner, Tracy. *Pregnancy and Childbirth.*

Kitzinger, Sheila. *The Experience of Childbirth.*

Chapter 7

Boston Women's Health Book Collective, The. *Our Bodies, Ourselves: A Book By and For Women*, Simon and Schuster, New York, Revised Edition, 1976.

Hewlett & Packard Medical Electronics, pamphlet. *You, Your Baby and Obstetrical Monitoring*, Copyright 1973, Printed in U.S.A.

Hotchner, Tracy. *Pregnancy & Childbirth: A Complete Guide For a New Life*, Avon Books, New York, 1979.

Tucker, Susan M., R.N., B.S.N. *Fetal Monitoring and Fetal Assessment in High-Risk Pregnancy*, The C. V. Mosby Co., St. Louis, Missouri, 1978.

Chapter 8

Brinkley, Ginny, Goldberg, Linda, and Kukar, Janice. *Your Child's First Journey*, Wayne, New Jersey: Avery Publishing Group Inc., 1982.

Hassid, Patricia. *Textbook for Childbirth Educators*, Maryland, New York: Harper & Row, 1978.

Kitzinger, Sheila. *The Complete Book of Pregnancy and Childbirth*.

Noble, Elizabeth. *Essential Exercising for the Childbearing Year: A Guide to Health and Comfort Before and After Your Baby is Born*. Boston: Houghton–Mifflin, 1976.

Chapter 9

Awake and Aware: Participating in Childbirth Through Psychoprophylaxis, Irwin Chabon, New York, Dell Publishing, 1966, p. 160.

Birth: Facts and Legends, Caterine Nilinaire, New York, Harmony Books, 1974, p. 304.

Birth Without Violence, Frederich Leboyer, New York, Alfred A. Knopf, 1976, p. 114.

The Cesarean Birth Experience: A Practical Comprehensive and Reassuring Guide for Parents and Professionals, updated version, Boston, Beacon, 1978, p. 241.

Childbirth: A Manual for Pregnancy and Delivery, John Seldon Miller, New York, Atheneum, 1971, p. 172.

Childbirth Today: Prepared and Positive, Carol Thompson, Dallar, Family Life Information Centre, 1978, p. 246.

Choices in Childbirth, Silvia Feldman, New York, Grosset & Dunlap, 1978, p. 246.

Commonsense Childbirth, Lester Dessey Hazell, New York, Berkley Publishing, 1969, p. 281.

The Course and Conduct of Normal Labor and Delivery, Keith Russell, M.D., pp. 565-593.

Creative Fitness for Baby and Child, Suzy Prudden and Leffrey Sussman, New York, William Morrow, 1972, p. 160.

Current Obstetric and Gynecology Diagnosis and Treatment, Ralph C. Benson, M.D., 1976, ch. 31.

Essential Exercising for the Childbearing Year: A Guide to Health and Comfort Before and After Your Baby is Born, Elizabeth Noble, Boston, Houghton-Mifflin, 1976, p. 180.

Human Reproduction: The Cone Content of Obstetrics, Gynecology and Perineal Medicine, 2nd Ed., Ernest W. Page, M.D., Claude A. Willee, M.D., ch. 14, pp. 284-320.

The New Childbirth, Erna Wright, New York, Pocket Books, 1971, p. 205.

Pregnancy in Anatomical Illustrations, Carnation Co., Ltd., Toronto, Carnation Co., 1971, p. 23.

Preparation for Childbirth: A Lamaze Guide, Donna Ewry and Roger Ewry, 2nd ed., New York, Signet Books, 1976, p. 224.

Prepared Childbirth, Tarvez Tucker, Dell Publishing Co., Inc., July 1981, p. 180.

Six Practical Lessons for an Easier Childbirth, Elizabeth Bing, rev. ed., Toronto, Bantam Books, 1977, p. 138.

Chapter 10

Awake and Aware: Participating in Childbirth Through Psychoprophylaxis, Irwin Chabon, New York, Dell Publishing, 1966, p. 160.

Birth: Facts and Legends, Caterine Nilinaire, New York, Harmony Books, 1974, p. 304.

Birth Without Violence, Frederich Leboyer, New York, Alfred A. Knopf, 1976, p. 114.

Bibliography

The Cesarean Birth Experience: A Practical Comprehensive and Reassuring Guide for Parents and Professionals, updated version, Boston, Beacon, 1978, p. 241.

Childbirth: A Manual for Pregnancy and Delivery, John Seldon Miller, New York, Atheneum, 1971, p. 172.

Childbirth Today: Prepared and Positive, Carol Thompson, Dallar, Family Life Information Centre, 1978, p. 246.

Choices in Childbirth, Silvia Feldman, New York, Grosset & Dunlap, 1978, p. 246.

Commonsense Childbirth, Lester Dessey Hazell, New York, Berkley Publishing, 1969, p. 281.

The Course and Conduct of Normal Labor and Delivery, Keith Russell, M.D., pp. 565-593.

Creative Fitness for Baby and Child, Suzy Prudden and Leffrey Sussman, New York, William Morrow, 1972, p. 160.

Current Obstetric and Gynecology Diagnosis and Treatment, Ralph C. Benson, M.D., 1976, ch. 31.

Essential Exercising for the Childbearing Year: A Guide to Health and Comfort Before and After Your Baby is Born, Elizabeth Noble, Boston, Houghton-Mifflin, 1976, p. 180.

Human Reproduction: The Cone Content of Obstetrics, Gynecology and Perineal Medicine, 2nd Ed., Ernest W. Page, M.D., Claude A. Willee, M.D., ch. 14, pp. 284-320.

The New Childbirth, Erna Wright, New York, Pocket Books, 1971, p. 205.

Pregnancy in Anatomical Illustrations, Carnation Co., Ltd., Toronto, Carnation Co., 1971, p. 23.

Preparation for Childbirth: A Lamaze Guide, Donna Ewry and Roger Ewry, 2nd ed., New York, Signet Books, 1976, p. 224.

Prepared Childbirth, Tarvez Tucker, Dell Publishing Co., Inc., July 1981, p. 180.

Six Practical Lessons for an Easier Childbirth, Elizabeth Bing, rev. ed., Toronto, Bantam Books, 1977, p. 138.

Chapter 11

Arms, Suzanne. *Immaculate Deception*. Houghton–Mifflin Company, Boston, 1975.

Bardwick, J. M., 1971. *Psychology of Women: A Study of Biocultural Conflicts*, New York: Harper & Row Publishers, Inc.

Bing, Elizabeth. *Six Practical Lessons for an Easier Childbirth*.

Bradley, R. A., 1974. Husband-Coached Childbirth, 2nd Edition. New York: Harper and Row, Publishers, Inc.

Casserley, Norman. "I, Midwife," *Prevention*. July, 1973, pp. 107-114.

Chabon, Irwin. *Awake and Aware*.

Dick-Read, Grantly. *Childbirth Without Fear*. New York, Edition 19.

Dwyer, J. M., 1976. *Human Reproduction: The Female System and The Neonate*, Philadelphia: F. A. Davis Co.

Guttmacher, Alan. *Pregnancy, Birth and Family Planning*.

Karmel, Marjorie. *Thank You, Dr. Lamaze*.

Kitzinger, Sheila. *The Experience of Childbirth*. London: Victor Collancz, 1962.

Kitzinger, Sheila. *Giving Birth*. Schocken Books, 1977 Edition, U.S.A.

Lamaze, Fernand. *Painless Childbirth*. Pocket Book Edition, 1976, New York, U.S.A.

Leboyer, F. *Birth Without Violence*.

McBride, A. B. *The Growth and Development of Mothers*.

Myles, Margaret. *Textbook for Midwives*, London.

Olds, Sally B. *et al. Nursing*, Addison-Wesley Publishing Company. California, 1980.

Chapter 13

Awake and Aware: Participating in Childbirth Through Psychoprophylaxis, Irwin Chabon, New York, Dell Publishing, 1966, p. 160.

Birth: Facts and Legends, Caterine Nilinaire, New York, Harmony Books, 1974, p. 304.

Birth Without Violence, Frederick Leboyer, New York, Alfred A. Knopf, 1976, p. 114.

The Cesarean Birth Experience: A Practical Comprehensive and Reassuring Guide for Parents and Professionals, updated version, Boston, Beacon, 1978, p. 241.

Childbirth: A Manual for Pregnancy and Delivery, John Seldon Miller, New York, Atheneum, 1971, p. 172.

Childbirth Today: Prepared and Positive, Carol Thompson, Dallar, Family Life Information Centre, 1978, p. 246.

Choices in Childbirth, Silvia Feldman, New York, Grosset & Dunlap, 1978, p. 246.

Commonsense Childbirth, Lester Dessey Hazell, New York, Berkley Publishing, 1969, p. 281.

The Course and Conduct of Normal Labor and Delivery, Keith Russell, M.D., pp. 565-593.

Creative Fitness for Baby and Child, Suzy Prudden and Leffrey Sussman, New York, William Morrow, 1972, p. 160.

Current Obstetric and Gynecology Diagnosis and Treatment, Ralph C. Benson, M.D., 1976, ch. 31.

Essential Exercising for the Childbearing Year: A Guide to Health and Comfort Before and After Your Baby is Born, Elizabeth Noble, Boston, Houghton-Mifflin, 1976, p. 180.

Human Reproduction: The Cone Content of Obstetrics, Gynecology and Perineal Medicine, 2nd Ed., Ernest W. Page, M.D., Claude A. Willee, M.D., ch. 14, pp. 284-320.

The New Childbirth, Erna Wright, New York, Pocket Books, 1971, p. 205.

Pregnancy in Anatomical Illustrations, Carnation Co., Ltd., Toronto, Carnation Co., 1971, p. 23.

Preparation for Childbirth: A Lamaze Guide, Donna Ewry and Roger Ewry, 2nd ed., New York, Signet Books, 1976, p. 224.

Prepared Childbirth, Tarvez Tucker, Dell Publishing Co., Inc., July 1981, p. 180.

Six Practical Lessons for an Easier Childbirth, Elizabeth Bing, rev. ed., Toronto, Bantam Books, 1977, p. 138.

Chapter 14

Bromage, R. Philip, *Epidural Anesthesia*, Ayerst Laboratories, 1972.

Da Cruz, V., Burnett, C. W. F., *Baillieère's Midwives' Dictionary*, 5th Edition, Baillière Tindall and Cassell, London, 1969.

Field, P. A., "Relief of Pain in Labour," *The Canadian Nurse*, December, 1974, pp. 17-23.

Hassid, Patricia, *Textbook for Childbirth Educators*, Harper and Row, New York, 1978.

Kitzinger, S., *The Experience of Childbirth*, Middlesex, England, Pelican Books, 1977.

Lamaze, F., *Painless Childbirth*, Air Pocket Books, New York, 1972.

Read, G. D., *Childbirth Without Fear*, New York, Harper and Row, 1972.

Oxorn, H., Foote, W. R., *Human Labour and Birth*, Appleton-Century-Crofts, New York, 1964.

Steele, G. C., *Epidural Nerve Block in Obstetrics*, Nursing Mirror, April 19, 1974.

Chapter 17

Banter, R. H., 1968. "Induction of Labor; Helpful or Harmful?" *Post Grad. Med.* 43:141.

Cardano, A., and Kraus, V., 1972. "Clinical Experience with Oxytocin," *Obst. Gynecol.* 39:247.

Hon, E. A., 1976. *Fetal Monitoring During Induction of Labor* ed. Parke-Davis Company. Greenwich, Conn.: CPC Communication, Inc.

Chapter 18

Donovan, B. *The Cesarean Birth Experience.* Boston Press, 1978.

Meyer, L. D. *The Cesarean (R)evolution.* Washington: Chas Franklin Press, 1981.

Mitchell, K. and Nason, M. *Cesarean Birth.* San Francisco: Harbor Publishing, 1981.

Polomeno, V. "The Impact of Cesarean Section Birth on Fathers: A Descriptive Study." Montreal: unpublished Master's Nursing Paper, 1981.

Wainer Cohen, N. "Minimizing Emotional Sequellae of Cesarean Childbirth," *Birth and the Family Journal.* 4:3:114-119, Fall 1977.

Wilson, C. C. and Hovey, W. R. *Cesarean Childbirth: A Handbook for Parents.* New York: Doubleday and Co., 1980.

Chapter 19

Pregnancy, Birth & Family Planning, Dr. A. Guttmacher.

Textbook for Midwives, Margaret Miles.

What's New, Mary Lou Rozdilsky & Barbara Banet.

Chapter 20

Brinkley, Ginny; Goldberg, Linda; Kukar, Janice. *Your Child's First Journey*, Wayne, New Jersey: Avery Publishing Group Inc., 1982.

Kitzinger, Sheila. *The Complete Book of Pregnancy and Childbirth*, New York. Alfred A. Knopf, 1982.

Noble, Elizabeth. *Essential Exercises for the Childbearing Year*, Boston: Houghton–Mifflin Co., 1976.

Chapter 21

Breastfeeding After a Cesarean Birth, Ross Laboratories; Columbus, Ohio; 1972.

Breastfeeding and Working; Cahil, Mary Ann; La Leche League International, Inc.; Publication No. 58; Franklin Park, Illinois, 1976.

Breastfeeding Your Baby; Second Edition, revised and expanded by Walker, Marsha and Watson Driscoll, Jeanne; Wayne, New Jersey; Avery Publishing Group, Inc.; 1978.

The Complete Book of Breastfeeding; Eiger, Marvin S. and Wendkos Olds, Sally; Bantam Books, U.S.A.; 1972.

How the Maternity Nurse Can Help the Breastfeeding Mother; Countryman, Betty Ann; La Leche League International, Inc.; Publication No. 118; Franklin Park, Illinois; 1977.

Nursing Your Baby; Pryor, Karen; Paper Jacks Ltd.; Ontario, Canada, 1973.

Chapter 22

The Complete Book of Breastfeeding; Eiger, Marvin S., M.D. and Olds, Sally Wendkos; Workman Publishing Company, Inc.; New York; 1972.

Current Knowledge on Breastfeeding; Psiaki, Donna and Olson, Christine; Division of Nutritional Sciences; Cornell University; 1977.

Feeding Your Child; Lambert, Lagacé, Louise; Ampersard Pub. Services Inc.; Toronto; 1976.

Freezing Breastmilk at Home; Theberge, Rousselet, Denyse; The Canadian Nurse; March, 1976.

The Modern Management of Successful Breast Feeding, Applebaum, R. M.; Pediatric Clinics of North America, Vol. 17, No. 1; 1970.

Nursing Your Baby; Pryor, Karen; Pocket Books; New York; 1973.

Nutrition and Diet Therapy; Williams, Sue Rodwell; C. V. Mosby Company; Saint Louis; 1977.

Chapter 23

Babyhood; Leach, Penelope; Penguin Books; Great Britain.

Caring for the Baby; Partridge, James; St. Paul's House; London, England; 1975.

Exercises for Your Baby; Lévy, Janine; William Collins, Sons and Company, Ltd.; Great Britain; 1973.

The Experience of Childbirth; Kitzinger, Sheila; Penguin Books; Markham, Ontario; 1978.

The First Twelve Months of Life; Caplan F.; Bantam Books, Toronto; 1978.

Infant Feeding; Gunther, Mavis; Penguin Books; Chauser Press; Middlesex, England; 1973.

A Lamaze Manual for Prepared Childbirth and Infant Care; Carr, Marcia Hirano and Jankowski, Joan LeBrecht; Avery Publishing Group Inc.; New Jersey, 1980.

Maternal Infant Bonding; Klaus, M.; Kennel, J.

Nursing Your Baby; Pryor, Karen; Kangaroo Books; Simon and Schuster; New York; 1973.

Pregnancy and Childbirth; Hutchner, Tracy.

Six Practical Lessons for an Easier Childbirth; Bing, Elizabeth; Bantam Books, Toronto.

Chapter 24

Kennel, J. H., Slyter, H., Klaus, M.: "The Mourning Response of Parents to the Death of a Newborn Infant." *N. Engl. J. Med.* 2?3: 344-349, 1970.

La Roche, Catherine *et. al.* "Grief Reaction to Perinatal Death: An Exploratory Study." *Psychosomatics* Vol 23 - No. 5, 1982.

La Roche, Catherine *et. al.* "Grief Reaction to Perinatal Death: A Follow–Up Study." *Can. Journal of Psychiatry* Vol 29 Feb., 1984.

Lockwood, S., Lewis, I. C. "Management of Grieving After Stillbirth." *Med. Journal. Australia*, 1980: 2 308-11.

Chapter 25

Guttmacher, Alan F. *Pregnancy, Birth and Family Planning.*

Manisoff, Miriem T. *Family Planning.*

Montreal Planned Parenthood Association.

Povey, W. G. *A Guide to Family Planning.*

Index

Abdomen, 9, 79, 92, 99
Abdominal tightening, 46, 102, 117, 119
Abnormal bleeding tendencies, 75
Abruptio placenta, 92
Accelerated-decelerated breathing, 68, 69, 78
Active labour, 58, 61-62, 68, 78, 83, 89
Adductor stretch, 45
Admitting office, 77, 107
Afterbirth. *See* Placenta, delivery of.
Afterpains, 112
Alcohol, 21
Alphafetoprotein, 37
Alveoli, 124, 125
Ambivalent feelings, 25
Ambulation, 113
Amniocentesis, 35-37, 93
Amnionhook, 88
Amniotic fluid, 7, 35-37, 58-59, 100
Amniotic sac, 57, 58, 61, 92, 99. *See also* Membranes.
Analgesics, 5, 101, 113
Anatomy
   cervix, 6, 8, 33
   pelvic floor, 6, 70, 117
   pelvis, 58
   perineum, 63, 73, 89, 91, 114, 120
   uterus, 6, 7, 53
   vagina, 6, 7, 65, 72, 75, 76, 90, 94, 107
Anencephalus, 35, 37
Anesthesia, 5, 73, 92
   epidural, 5, 74-76, 89, 98, 101, 107
   general, 5, 98, 101, 107
   local, 5, 73, 86, 89, 90, 101
   paracervical, 5, 73
   pudendal, 5, 74, 89
Anesthesiologist, 73, 74, 75, 76, 97

Anger, and pain response, 104
Ankle rotating, 102
Antepartum hemorrhage, 75, 88, 91, 92
Antibiotics, 92
Antibodies, 121
Anxiety, 3, 72, 76, 85, 126
Apgar rating, 63, 134
Apprehension, 76, 82
Areola, 8, 124
Arm stretch, 44
Artificial rupture of membranes, 4, 82, 88
Assessment of newborn, 100, 134
Asthma, 88

B-Scan. *See* Ultrasound.
Baby
   appearance at birth, 100, 134
   bathing, 65, 142
   birth of, 134. *See also* Labour and delivery.
   burping, 103, 128-129
   care of, 134-144
   constipation, 121, 137
   cord care, 5, 137, 142
   death of, 145-146
   equipment for, 139, 142-143. *See also* Layette.
   feeding, 5, 100, 103, 121-129, 130-133
   immunizations, 5, 142
   jaundice, 123, 136
   lanugo, 26, 139
   meconium, 125, 138
   reflexes, 140-141
   safety, 5
   senses, 5
   skin, 5, 139
   sleep, 5, 139, 140

umbilical cord stump, 5, 137, 142
vernix, 26, 134
vision, 5, 141
weaning, 5, 129
weight, changes in, 36, 65
Back
   ache, 26, 41, 49, 75, 84, 117
   care, 41, 82
   labour, 59, 78, 79, 81, 83, 87
   pressure, 87
Bag of waters, 57, 58, 61, 92, 99. *See also* Membranes.
Bartholin's glands, 7
Bearing down. *See* Pushing.
Bent leg lift, 47, 119
Bikini incision (Pfannenstiel), 98
Bilirubin, 35, 136
Birth canal, 89
Birth control, 115, 147-152
Bladder, 6, 98, 112
Bleeding
   antepartum, 75, 88, 91, 92
   postpartum, 100, 111
Blood
   tests, 33, 35, 96
   type, 33, 96
   volume, 9, 26, 112
Blood pressure, 33, 60, 65, 75, 88, 96, 97
Bloody show, 8, 25, 31, 57, 58, 81-84
"Blue" tinge, 63
Blurring of vision, 71
Body changes during pregnancy, 24-26
Body mechanics, 41-43
Bonding, 63, 115, 128
Bottle feeding, 130-133
Bowel movement
   baby, 5, 121, 122, 137-138
   postpartum, 114
   during pregnancy, 22
Braxton-Hicks contractions, 7, 26, 57, 81
Breasts
   of baby, 136
   changes during pregnancy, 6, 8, 124, 125
   and milk production, 111, 113, 121, 125
Breastfeeding
   advantages, 22, 111, 121
   colostrum, 8, 25, 113, 125
   and contraception, 115, 121
   on the delivery table, 80, 86, 107, 128
   engorgement, 113, 125, 127
   father's role, 106, 121, 124
   fluid intake, 113
   hormones, 113, 121, 123, 125, 126, 136
   menstrual cycle, 115, 121, 125
   nursing bras, 113, 127
   and the pediatrician, 107, 130
   postcesarean, 100, 103, 106, 122-123
   and premature babies, 122-123
   and sexual relations, 31, 122
   and suppression of lactation, 113
   uterine contractions during, 112, 126
Breastmilk, 121, 122, 129
Breech presentation, 4, 89, 90, 91
Breathing techniques
   benefits, 3, 4, 39, 66, 77, 103
   patterns, 61, 62, 68, 69, 78, 79, 83, 89

Caffeine, 19-20, 129
Calcium, 9
Camomile tea, 140
Car seat, 143
Cardiac disease, 88, 90, 93
Catheter, urinary, 98, 102, 107
Cephalo-pelvic disproportion (C.P.D.), 4, 35, 88, 89, 90, 96
Cervix
   changes, 6, 8, 33
   dilatation, 57, 58, 62, 70, 72, 79, 89
   effacement, 57, 82, 83
   See also Bloody show.
Cesarean baby, 101, 105
Cesarean birth, 92-108
   anesthesia, 92, 98, 101-102
   emergency, 92, 96, 105
   exercise after, 102, 120
   father-attended, 78, 96, 98, 104, 105, 107
   incisions, 98, 103
   indications for, 40, 92
   planned, 92, 96
   postpartum, 31, 80, 102-103, 106-107
Chadwick's sign, 7
Chromosomes, 11
Circumcision, 137
Classical incision, 98
Cleansing breath, 53, 54, 63, 68, 70, 79, 80, 83, 85
Clips (Michel), 100, 103
Coach. *See* Father; Partner.
Coach's reminder sheet, 77-80
Coitus interruptus (withdrawal method), 147, 150
Colic, 140
Colostrum, 8, 25, 113, 125
Combined pattern, 68, 69, 79, 83
Comfort measures in labour, 68
Concentration, 66, 67, 84, 89
Conditioned reflexes, 3, 53-54
Conditioning exercises, 44-48, 66, 117-120
Condom, 147, 149
Consent forms, 97
Constipation
   baby, 121, 137
   postpartum, 114
   during pregnancy, 22
Contraception, 115, 147-152
Contractions
   afterpains, 112-113
   Braxton-Hicks, 7, 26, 57, 81

labour, 3, 39, 53, 57, 58, 59, 61, 68, 70, 72, 76, 78, 79, 82-86, 88, 89, 92, 96
   timing of, 77, 82
Control, 68, 77
Controlled relaxation
   defined, 53-54
   exercises for, 4, 55-56
Cord compression, 94
Counterpressure, 78, 83, 84, 87
Cow's milk, 131
Cradle cap, 135
Cramps, in calves and toes, 49
Creams and foams, 147, 151
Cribs, 63, 86, 134
Crying in newborns, 139

Death of baby, 145-146
Deep chest breathing, 68, 69, 79, 80
Delivery
   of baby, 72, 85, 90
   forceps, 4, 89, 90, 91, 94
   of placenta, 58, 63, 73, 86, 100, 111, 113, 134
Delivery room, 5, 80
Demerol, 101
Depression, postpartum, 105
Diabetes, 88, 93
Diagnostic tests and procedures, 33-40, 93
Diaper rash, 136
Diapers, 138
Diaphragm, 147, 150
Diarrhea, 137
Diastasis recti, 47, 119
Dilatation, 57, 58, 62, 70, 72, 79, 89
Disappointment, 104
Disc disease, 75
Discipline, 66, 67
Dizziness, 71
Douching, 150, 151
Drowsiness, 84, 85
Drugs. *See* Medications.

Early labour, 57-59, 77-78, 82
Eclampsia. *See* Pre-eclampsia.
Edema, 9, 26, 49, 96
Effacement, 57, 82, 83
Effleurage, 53, 61, 79, 83
Elective cesarean, 92, 96
Elective induction, 4, 88
Elimination, 138
Emotional changes, 81
Emotional support during labour, 77-80
Encouragement, 82, 83, 84, 105
Enema
   labour, 88
   postoperative, 103
   postpartum, 114
Energy, 18, 53, 72, 81

Engagement, 58, 89
Engorgement, 113, 114, 125, 127
Epidural anesthesia, 5, 74-76, 89, 98, 101
Epilepsy, 88
Episiotomy, 4, 63, 73, 85, 86, 89, 90, 112 113-114
Estriol level, 35, 40
Excitement, 25-26, 65, 82, 85, 86
Exercises
   body mechanics, 41-43
   breathing, 68-71
   cesarean, post-op, 102, 120
   conditioning, 44-48, 66, 117-120
   Kegel, 48
   postpartum, 114, 117-120
   posture, 41-43, 117
   prenatal, 3, 21, 44-48
   relaxation, 53, 56
Exhaustion. *See* Fatigue.
Expulsion
   of baby, 62, 72, 80, 85, 90
   of placenta, 58, 63, 73, 86, 100, 111, 113, 134
External fetal monitor, 4, 38-40, 61, 89, 94, 97

Facecloth, 83, 84, 87, 105
Failure, 72, 104
Fallopian tubes, 6, 7
False labour, 81
Family centred maternity care, 3, 104, 113
Family planning, 115, 147-152
Father, 27-29
   bonding, 27-29, 113, 115
   and cesarean birth, 78, 96, 98, 104, 105, 107
   feelings about sex, 30-31
   postpartum, 28, 113, 114, 115
   See also Partner.
Fatigue
   during labour, 72, 73, 84, 86, 89
   postpartum, 111, 112, 113, 114, 116
   during pregnancy, 25
Fear-tension-pain cycle, 72
Fears during pregnancy, 3, 26, 104
Female reproductive organs, 6-9
Female sterilization, 147, 152
Fetal
   anomalies, 35, 37
   development, 25
   distress, 4, 40, 89, 90, 91, 94
   heart monitor, 4, 38-40, 61, 89, 94, 97
   heart rate, 26, 59, 60, 62, 75, 88, 89, 97, 98
   movements, 59, 81
Fetal assessment. *See* Diagnostic tests and procedures.
Fetus, 7, 34, 58, 94
First stage of labour
   active labour, 58, 61-62, 68, 78, 83, 89
   early labour, 57-59, 77-78, 82
   transition, 58, 62, 79, 84
First trimester of pregnancy, 8, 25

Fluid intake, 113, 114
Fluoride, 16-17
Foam, contraceptive, 147, 151
Focal point, 53, 68, 79, 80, 83, 84
Folic acid, 17
Fontanelles, 135
Food groups, 20
Foods to avoid, 19
Forceps delivery, 4, 89, 90, 91, 94
Foremilk, 125
Fundal pressure, 100
Fundus, 89

Gas, 82, 103, 140
General anesthesia, 5, 98, 101, 107
German measles, 35
Grasp reflex, 140
Grieving process, 145-146
Gripe water, 140
Gums, 25

Hand expression of milk, 122, 126
Headache, 82, 101
Heartburn (indigestion), 22, 26, 140
Heat lamp, 114
Heat loss, in newborn baby, 139
Hemorrhage, antepartum, 88, 92
Hemorrhoids, 49, 114, 115
Herpes virus, 93
Hiccups, 84
Hind-milk, 125
Hip bones, 58
HMD, 37
Hormones
    breastfeeding, 113, 121, 125, 126, 136
    oxytocin, 39, 86, 89, 96, 97, 100, 111, 126
    prolactin, 113, 125
Hospital, 59-60, 81, 107, 111
    and family centred care, 3, 104, 113
Hyaline membrane syndrome (HMD), 37
Hydramnios, 35
Hydrocephaly, 35
Hypertension, 88, 96
Hyperventilation
    and leg cramps, 9
    prevention of, 81, 86
    in respiratory technique, 71
Hypotension, maternal, 75, 97, 101

Ice chips, 84
Identification bands, 63
Immunizations, 142-143
Incision
    cesarean, 98, 103
    episiotomy, 4, 63, 73, 85, 86, 89, 90, 112, 113-114
Incubator, 63, 135
Indigestion, 22, 140

Induction of labour, 4, 88-89
Infection
    cesarean, 92, 96
    postpartum, 114, 115
Infertility, 88
Intercourse, 115
Intrauterine device (I.U.D.), 147, 148-149
Intravenous fluids, 4, 5, 39, 89, 96, 97, 101, 102, 111
Inverted nipples. 127
Involution, 111
Iron, 97, 114
Irritability, 83, 84, 114
Ischial spines, 89
I.U.D. *See* Intrauterine device.

Jaundice, 123, 136

Kegel exercises, 48, 120
Kidney disease, 93

La Leche League, 103
Labour and delivery
    active labour, 58, 61-62, 68, 78, 83, 89
    anxiety about, 3, 72
    early labour, 57-59, 77-78, 82
    false labour, 57
    first stage, 57-59, 61-62, 68, 77-79, 82-84, 89
    induction of, 4, 88-89
    and medications, 72, 75, 76
    relaxation for, 72, 77-79, 81-84, 85
    second stage, 58, 75, 76, 79, 80-85, 89
    support during, 3, 4, 62, 68, 79, 82
    third stage, 58, 63, 86
    transition, 58, 62, 79, 84
    true labour signs, 57
Labour partner
    guidelines for, 81-87
    role of, 77-80
Lacerations, 63
Lamaze bag, 77, 78
Lanugo, 26, 139
Laxatives, 114
Layette, 143, 144. *See also* Baby, equipment for.
Leg cramps, 9, 84
Leg sliding, 118
Lesions, 93
Let-down reflex, 122, 125, 126
Ligaments, 6, 7
Lightening, 26, 81
Linea nigra, 26
Local anesthetic, 5, 73, 86, 89, 90, 101
Lochia, 65, 102, 103, 112, 113
Lordosis, 41
Losing a baby, 145-146
L/S ratio (lecithin/sphingomyelin ratio), 37
Lung disease, 93

Male reproductive organs, 10-11
Male sterilization, 147, 151-152
Malpresentation, 94
Mask of pregnancy, 26
Massage
    labour, 61, 83
    to relieve "backache labour," 87
    in touch relaxation, 61
Maternal-infant bonding, 128
Meconium, 4, 37, 94, 125, 138
Medical history, 32
Medications
    during labour, 73, 74-75, 76, 79
    post-operative, 102, 103, 106
    during pregnancy, 21
    pre-operative, 97, 107
Membranes
    artificial rupture of, 4, 82, 88
    intact, 57, 61, 92
    rupture of, 4, 57, 58-59, 82, 89, 94, 96
Menstrual cycle, 32, 82, 147-148
    postpartum, 115, 121, 125
Menu samples, 20
Metric measures, 23
Milia, 139
Miscarriage, 36, 88
Modified deep chest breathing, 68, 69, 79
Montgomery's glands, 8, 25, 124
Moodiness, 10, 25, 84
Morning sickness, 21-22
Moro reflex, 141
Morphine, 101, 102
Mourning a baby, 145-146
Mucus plug. *See* Bloody show.
Multiple birth, 88, 90, 95
Multiple pregnancy. *See* Multiple birth.
Multiple sclerosis, 75

Narcotics, 73
Nausea, 21-22, 25, 84
Neural tube defect, 37
Neurological disease, 75, 101
Neuromuscular control, 53
Nipples, 126-127
Nitrous oxide, 73, 76, 101
Non-stress test, 39, 93
Numbness, 9, 49, 75
Nursery, 80, 134
Nutrition
    baby, 12-23, 129
    daily menu samples, 20
    and energy, 18-19
    food groups, chart, 20
    food guide, 14-16
    during lactation, 22-23, 115, 129, 131
    nutrient composition, chart, 12
    during pregnancy, 12-23
    snacking, 19, 115
    special needs, 18
    supplements, 17

Obstetrician, 4, 73, 88, 89, 94, 105
Occipito posterior position. *See* Posterior position.
OCT. *See* Oxytocin challenge test.
Onset of labour, 57-59, 77, 82
Operating room, 5, 78, 80, 97, 107
Oral contraceptives, 147-148
Ovaries, 6, 7, 125
Overdue baby, 88
Ovulation, 7, 121, 125
Oxytocin, 39, 86, 89, 96, 97, 100, 111, 126. *See also* Syntocinon.
Oxytocin challenge test (OCT), 39

Pacifier, 139
Pain, 3, 72, 92, 102, 103
Palpation, 92, 111
Panic, 79
Paracervical block, 5, 73
Partner, 3, 4
    at the birth, 28, 66, 81
    at cesarean birth, 98, 104, 105-106, 107
    emotional reactions of, 28-31, 104-105, 114, 115
    helping in the home, 29, 106, 142
    as parent, 28, 115, 142
    and prenatal classes, 28, 76, 104
    reminders for, 77-80
    support of, in labour, 3, 28, 38, 53-54, 62, 66-67, 68, 77-80, 81-87, 106
Paternal-infant bonding, 27-29, 113, 115
Pavlov, 66
Pectoral exercise, 45, 117, 120
Pediatrician, 5, 107, 142
Pelvic examinations
    antepartum, 33, 59, 62, 63, 79, 88
    postpartum, 115
Pelvic floor
    during delivery, 82, 85
    muscles, 6, 70, 117
Pelvic rock, 83, 78, 87
Pelvic tilt, 41, 46, 49, 117
    in 4-point kneel, 48
    in standing position, 118
Pelvis, 58
Penis, 10
Peppermint tea, 140
Perineal care, 114
Perineum, 63, 73, 89, 90, 91, 114, 120
Pfannenstiel incision, 98
Photography, 80, 107
Physical changes in labour, 81, 89
Placenta
    abruptio, 92
    delivery of, 58, 63, 73, 86, 100, 111, 113, 134

function of, 25
and hormones, 35
and pregnancy, 7, 34
previa, 92
Positions
during birth, 5, 62-63
during labour, 5, 61, 78, 80
Posterior position, 78, 89
Postmaturity, 88
Postpartum period, 31, 80, 109-152
cesarean, 106-107
and depression, 114
exercises, 114, 117-120
physical changes, 111, 114
Posture, 41, 44, 49, 117
Praise, 77, 80, 85, 86
Pre-eclampsia, 88, 90, 96
Pregnancy, 1-49
Premature baby, 89, 90, 134
Premature urge to push, 62, 79, 84
blowing out, 62, 79, 84
Prenatal testing, 33, 35-37, 93
Prepping, 107
Progesterone, 33, 125
Prolactin, 113, 125
Prolapsed cord, 94
Protein, 10, 96, 114
Pseudomenstruation, 137
Psychoprophylaxis, 3, 66, 72
Pudendal block, 5, 74, 89
Pushing, 62, 70, 79, 80, 84, 85
breathing patterns, 61, 62, 68, 69, 78, 79, 83, 89
positions, 5, 62-63

Quickening, 26

RDS. *See* Respiratory distress syndrome.
Reassurance, 77, 82, 83, 84
Recovery room, 80, 102, 107, 134
Recti muscles, 47, 119
Rectum, 6, 84, 85
Reflexes in baby, 140, 141
Regional anesthesia, 98, 100, 101, 107
Relatives, 78
Relaxation
during birth, 85
controlled, 66, 68
during labour, 72, 77-79, 81-84
techniques, 4, 39, 53-54, 59, 68, 72, 79, 81, 82
and touch, 61, 105
Repeated puff blows, 69, 79, 84
Reproductive organs
female, 6-9
female, changes after childbirth, 111, 112, 113, 127-128
male, 10-11

Resentment/anger, 104
Respiratory distress syndrome (RDS), 37
Response to stimulus, 66
Rest, 112
Rh incompatibility, 35, 88
Rhythm method of contraception, 147, 150-151
Rooming-in, 107
Rooting reflex, 141
Rubella, 35
Rupture of membranes
artificial, 4, 82, 88
spontaneous, 57, 58-59, 88, 89, 96

Sacrum, 58, 83
Salt, 9, 19
Scalp, fetal blood sample, 40
Sciatica, 75
Scrotum, 10
Scrub suit, 77
Second stage of labour, 58, 75, 76, 79, 80-85, 89
Second trimester of pregnancy, 26
Sedatives, 73
Self-image, 3, 26 30
Semen, 10
Seminal vesicles, 10
Seminiferous tubules, 10
Sex
of baby, 31
postpartum, 31, 106, 122
pregnancy, 25, 30-31
Shallow chest breathing, 61, 62, 68, 69
with puff blows, 68, 70, 79, 84
Shaving pubic hair, 88, 97
Shock/surprise, 105
Shoe covers, 77
Shortness of breath, 10, 26, 49
Show, 8, 25, 31, 57, 58, 81-84
Siblings, 106
Sickle cell anemia, 35
Sidelying position, 43
Signs of labour, 57
Sit-ups, 46-47, 119
Sitz bath, 114
Skin, 9
infant's, 26
Sleep
baby's, 5, 139, 140
and labour, 84
postpartum, 65, 112, 114
Smoking, 21
Soft spots, 135
Solid food, 132, 140
Sperm, 10
Spermatic cord, 10
Spermicides, 147, 151
Spina bifida, 37
Spinal anesthesia, 101
Spitting up, 128-129

Index

Spurt of energy, 81, 85
Stages of labour
    first, 57-59, 61-62, 68, 77-79, 82-84, 89
    second, 58, 75, 76, 79, 80-85, 89
    third, 58, 63, 86
Staples, 100, 103
Startle reflex, 141
Sterilizing bottles, 130
Stillbirth, 145-146
Stirrups, 62, 90
Stitches, 103, 113
Stress test, 39
Stretch marks. *See* Striae.
Striae, 9, 26
Sucking, 127, 128, 141
Suctioning of baby, 86, 100
Suitcases, 59-60
Supine hypotension, 75
Supine position, 43
Support person. *See* Partner.
Suppositories, 103
Sutures, (self-absorbent), 63, 100, 103, 113
Swelling, 9, 26, 49, 96
Symphysis pubis, 111
Syntocinon, 63. *See also* Oxytocin.

Tailbone, 58
Tailor stretch, 45
Temperature, 65, 97, 139
Tension, 53, 72
Testes, 10, 137
Third stage of labour, 58, 63, 86
Third trimester of pregnancy, 26
Thrush, 136
Thyroid gland, 25
Timing of contractions, 77, 82
Tingling, 9, 49, 75
Tiredness, 65, 85, 111
Touch relaxation, 61, 105
Toxemia of pregnancy, 96. *See also* Pre-eclampsia.
Tranquillizers, 5
Transducer, 38
Transition, 58, 62, 79, 84
Transverse presentation, 95
Trembling of extremities, 84
Trimesters of pregnancy
    first, 8, 25
    second, 26
    third, 26
Trunk reach, 44
Tubal ligation, 152
Twins, 88, 90, 95, 123

Ultrasound, 33, 93
Umbilical cord, 63, 86, 94, 137, 142

Umbilicus, mother's, 9, 26
Unmedicated childbirth, 72
Urethra, 10
Urge to push. *See* Pushing.
Urinary estriol test, 40
Urinary infection, 33
Urination
    baby's, 138
    during labour, 78
    postpartum, 89, 102, 112
    during pregnancy, 25, 49
Urine tests, 33, 96
Uterine dystocia, 96
Uterus
    contractions of. *See* Contractions.
    incisions, 99
    postpartum, 65, 89
    during pregnancy, 6, 7, 53

Vaccinations
    infant's, 5, 142-143
    during pregnancy, 35
Vagina, 6, 7, 65, 72, 75, 76, 90, 94, 107
    discharge from, 94, 102, 103, 112, 113
    examination of, 33, 59, 62, 63, 79, 88, 115
    secretions of, 7, 25, 30, 81, 107
    tear in, 63, 90, 91
Varicose veins, 9, 26, 49
Vasectomy, 151-152
Venereal disease, 93
Verbal cues, 53, 62, 66, 68, 78
Vernix caseosa, 26, 134
Vertex presentation, 89
Vision, 5, 141
Visiting hours, 108
Vital signs, 65, 89, 97, 102
Vitamin D, 17
Voiding, 78, 83
Vomiting, 84
Vulva, 63, 113, 137

Water retention, 9, 10
Weaning, 129
Weight
    of baby, 136
    postpartum, 115
    during pregnancy, 10, 26
Withdrawal reflex, 141
Working and breastfeeding, 122

Xylocaine, 74